Fit Kids for Life:
A Parent's Guide to
Raising Healthy Children

by
Brandon McIntosh
and
Chrisoula Kiriazis, M.D.

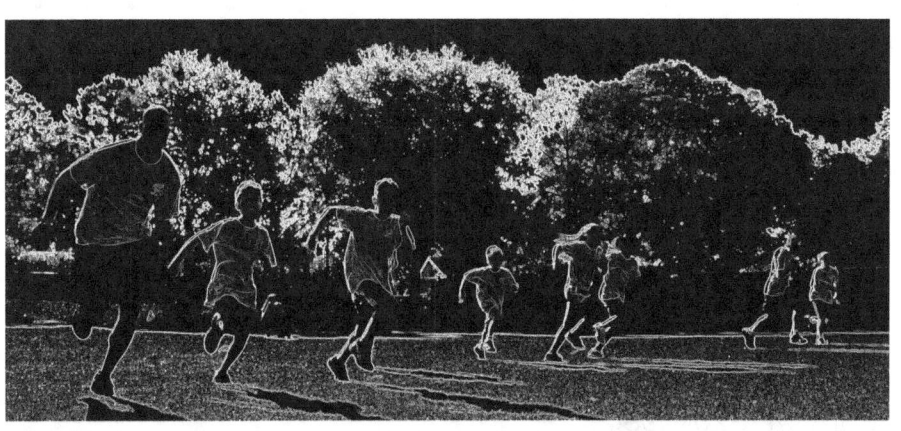

This book is dedicated to my family: Shirley, my dear mother, Danielle and Cameron, my sister and nephew. To my New Balance Tampa family, thank you for all your support. Thank you Dr. Kiriazis, for your vision and motivation in making this dream come true.

Brandon McIntosh

This book is dedicated to my husband, Winchester Dermody, my sons, Winchester and Zachary, and our dog, Kobi. They are the sun in my universe. To my husband, for taking all but one of the pictures in this book and being on call as my tech support guru, I love you. To my patients who make changes and get healthier, you make me excited to go to work every day.

Chrisoula Kiriazis, MD

FIT KIDS FOR LIFE: A PARENT'S GUIDE TO RAISING HEALTHY CHILDREN

Contents

WHY BE A FIT KID?

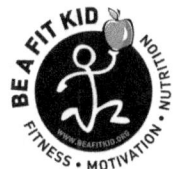

by Chrisoula Kiriazis M.D.

If you are reading this book, then you are ready to be part of a healthier America. You are ready to take action. You are overwhelmed by reading statistics about obesity, diabetes, and heart disease and you want your children to be active and healthy adults. You know that establishing good nutrition and exercise habits early in life is not optional but mandatory. Your kids may participate in lots of sports and activities but none of them teach your child about nutrition. You realize that giving your child a coach who is interested not only in physical training but in educating them about nutrition is a powerful force. The FITKIDS program is your secret weapon.

FITKIDS is a program that has been in place at the Southwest Recreation Center in Largo, Florida, since 2010, run by "KID WHISPERER" Brandon McIntosh. It consists of resistance and aerobic exercise in a group setting along with nutrition education using food logs. While there are similar programs throughout the country, this one is a notch above. How do I know that? I know that because I am a doctor with two boys, who have participated in martial arts, gymnastics, soccer, basketball, and flag football, and this is the FIRST and ONLY program my children have been part of that made them stronger, faster, more confident and got them talking about NUTRITION. They won't let me buy Oreos anymore! They have started cooking some meals! What happens in this FITKIDS program is so astounding to me that I felt compelled to write a book about it. I know that you and your children will be better for being part of FITKIDS. If you're not part of the program, this book is a good starting point to think about how you can make your family healthier.

CHAPTER ONE
YOUR AUTHORS

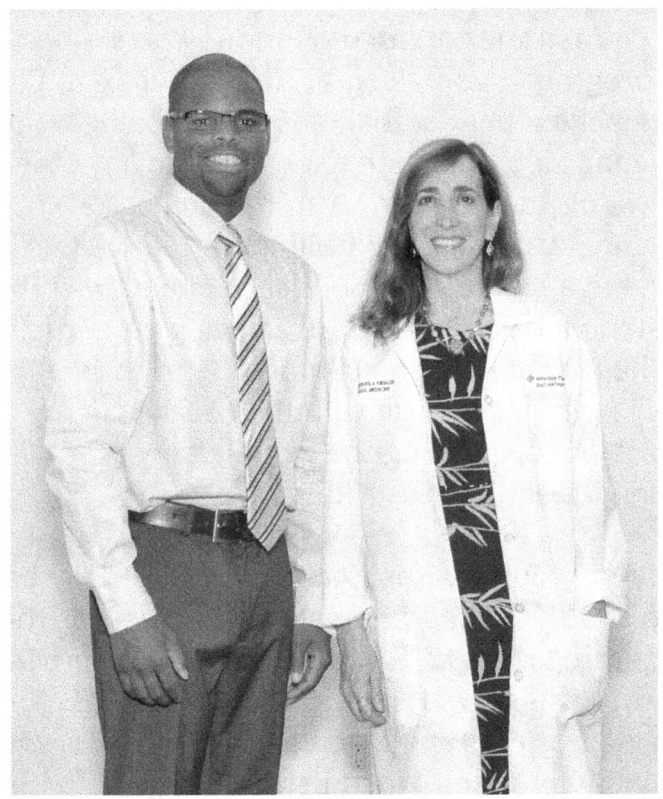

Brandon McIntosh, CPT

As a successful, college-educated, African-American male raised in a single-parent home, I have spent my whole life defying statistics. My mother worked hard to support my sister and me and always taught me to reach for my dreams. As a child, I fell in love with baseball and football and played throughout middle school and high school. I had a partial scholarship to go to college at Methodist University in Fayetteville, North Carolina, where I played football and got a bachelor's of science degree in sports management.. After graduating, I started working in baseball, including work with the Colorado Rockies and the Toronto Blue Jays. After almost five years, I decided that I needed to find my inspiration elsewhere. I wanted to work with kids.

The road led me to Largo, Florida, where I became recreation program supervisor at the Southwest Recreation Center. Coaching flag football and basketball gave me exposure to young kids who often hadn't played any other sports. I got to watch them progress from running down the field flapping their arms and stumbling over each other to being able to catch a football and run for a touchdown. These kids are invested in the game and are enjoying every moment. My role as their coach is to encourage them to play hard and never give up trying. Unlike with the coaches in my memory, my focus is not on winning the game at any cost but in helping children to achieve their best.

The other group of kids I got to see on a daily basis consisted of the kids doing aftercare at our facility. That was a different group. Most of those kids were not enrolled in any sports. They often lived in single-family homes. They dealt with challenging environments at home. Obesity was a common problem for them. When I started talking to these kids, I understood how much they were impacted by being overweight. Both boys and girls described being made fun of and being bullied because of their weight. They were embarrassed by their bodies and wore large clothes to cover themselves.

I started thinking about how I could help kids other than by coaching a sport. I could see that many of the kids around me were overweight. I knew the statistics for childhood obesity were bad. I saw firsthand the effect of diabetes on my mother and I wanted to make a difference. I knew that if I could defy statistics, so could these kids. I got certified as a personal trainer for children, nutrition specialist, and youth athletic performance specialist. I thought I could offer kids more by creating a program that helped them to get fit not only with exercise but by teaching them about nutrition. The idea for my version of FITKIDS developed as a natural consequence of all of these things. It is my way of help- ing to make the changes we need as a country if we want a healthier future. Change begins with each one of us and, for me, it begins with each of my kids and their families.

Thank you to Michelle Obama in Washington for making health and wellness in children a priority for America. In Florida, thank you to my boss, Joan Byrne, director of rec- reation for Largo, for supporting my vision of FITKIDS and helping me to get this program moving. Let's get fit!

Chrisoula Kiriazis, MD

As you may be able to tell from my name, I am a Greek girl. My parents got on a boat separately from Greece and met in Montreal, Quebec, Canada, where they raised my brother and me. My father is the original frugal barber and my mother worked as a maid until she got factory work for the duration of her working days. I was fortunate enough to go to medical school at McGill University, from which I graduated at age twenty-two. I fell in love with primary care medicine during my residency at North Shore Hospital in Manhasset, New York. For the last nineteen years, I've been a primary care physician at Morton Plant Mease Primary Care in Clearwater, Florida. I have had the privilege of knowing many families for years. Somewhere along the way, I was lucky enough to meet my husband and have two children.

Becoming a parent myself has been life-changing because I have another role to balance but it has also been incredibly fun.

As our journey through parenting has marched on, I have thought more about the effect of our lifestyles as parents on our children's health. When my kids got involved in FITKIDS, I became very excited that there was a program for children that incorporated a focus on both exercise and nutrition. Over the past two years, I have watched Brandon do amazing things with children, who are transformed because of it. Another piece of the puzzle is reaching parents. The program is more likely to be successful with parents who are actively involved. This book is the result of that need to engage parents in this program. My message is this: it doesn't take extraordinary measures to have healthy, active children who are at a normal weight. You don't have to enforce a sugar-free, vegetarian diet, your children don't need a personal trainer, and you don't need to be superhuman to organize it all. You do have to be conscious of what kind of food you are buying and eating, how much time you and your children are physically active, and how much screen time they use. As my favorite English teacher said many years ago, "With awareness comes change."

Why do we need to change?
- Seventeen percent of children aged two to nineteen are obese.
- Since 1980, the prevalence of childhood obesity has tripled.
- An obese child will often be an obese adult.
- More than 35 percent of American adults are obese.
- Obesity-related conditions include heart disease, stroke, and type-2 diabetes, as well as certain types of cancer, including breast cancer.

CHAPTER TWO
THE POWER OF EXERCISE

by Chrisoula Kiriazis, MD

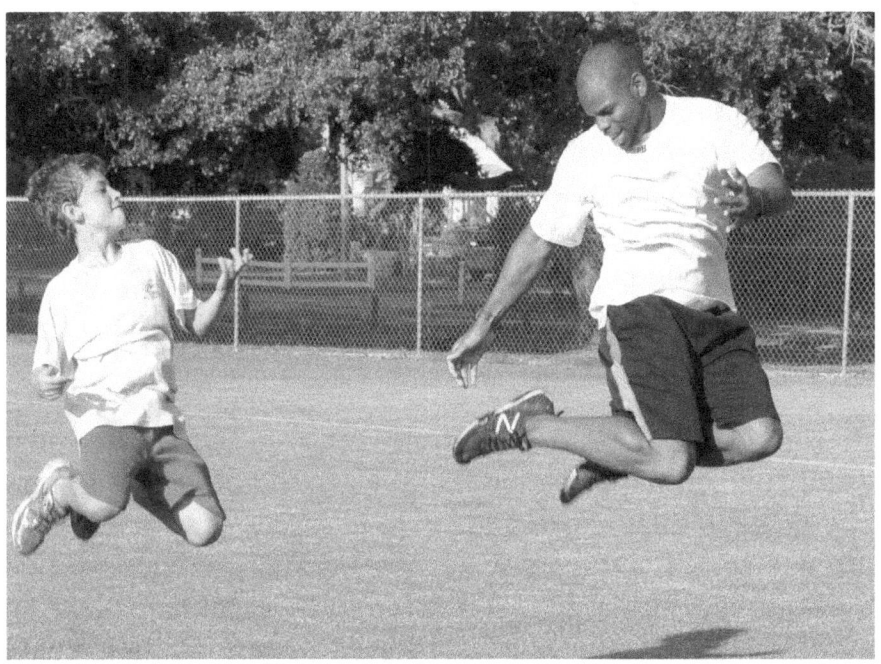

The benefits of exercise in children are tremendous. Let me list some important facts:

1. Children are less likely to be overweight or diabetic if they exercise regularly.
2. Exercise improves learning and academic performance. Is that why physical education is being taken out of most school schedules?
3. Exercise builds stronger bones and muscles.

4. Exercise improves mood and fosters self-confidence.
5. Children sleep more soundly and more easily when they exercise.

As I tell my patients, there is no pill that can offer the benefits of regular exercise. As our culture has moved from the outdoor to the indoor world, children have been exercising their fingers and eyes with screens more than other parts of their bodies. Also, children tend to classify themselves according to how they see themselves. A child who loves to read may perceive that he is a "bookworm." Another who likes computers may see herself as a "computer geek." These children may not perceive themselves as athletic or coordinated. A child who is overweight may feel he can't participate in competitive sports. These perceptions are reinforced if we allow children to avoid exercise. We know that exercise enhances learning so there is no reason for any child to avoid physical exertion. Children should be physically active for at least sixty minutes every day.

The way that children exercise has shifted. While most exercise used to happen in the playground or in a neighborhood, these days more and more exercise occurs in structured environments organized by adults. That has added a whole new arena of responsibility for parents. Where an evening in your childhood consisted of you coming home from school then going right outside until it was time to go home for dinner, the new schedule goes something like this: parents, who may or may not work, pick children up from school, drive to one or more activities (multiplied by the number of children), stop by the drive-through for dinner, and take the kids home to finish homework before collapsing for the night. For those parents who are too overwhelmed to do this, the alternative is a peaceful few hours while children sit in front of the TV, play video games, or browse on the computer. Most of us are guilty of using screens as babysitters.

The goal is to find balance in all things. It seems that we have high expectations of our children these days and also high expectations of ourselves as parents. Many children are introduced to organized sports at a young age. They may try a variety of sports, looking for one that they enjoy and are good at. There seems to be a focus on finding a competitive sport for children to excel in at a young age. Children often continue the same sport throughout their high school careers. That works well for some children but how about those children who do not excel in any particular sport? What message do they get? The message that we need to give them is this: exercise is an essential component of a healthy life. The goal is to exercise because it's good for you. It doesn't matter if you're not a star athlete. You don't have to go to the Olympics. You don't have to do the same activity every day. Trying different sports and activities is a great idea. You don't have to be fearless and you don't have to finish first. Be warned, however, that if you are active, you will FEEL GOOD AND HAVE FUN!

FITKIDS is a great way for a child to develop lifelong exercise habits without the pressure of having to win. Not all children enjoy the pressure of team sports(or their parents yelling loudly from the sidelines) but all children need to exercise. FITKIDS is not about winning but it is about striving. FITKIDS is about kids learning to be healthy but also having fun doing it. Kids get the opportunity to challenge themselves in a nurturing and inspiring environment. The result is that they usually exceed their expectations....

CHAPTER THREE
THE SCIENCE OF EXERCISE

by Chrisoula Kiriazis, MD

More and more research is emerging in the field of exercise physiology. While it may seem like common sense to say that exercise is healthy, looking at the actual mechanisms that lead to the benefits is fascinating.

How does exercise reduce the risk of obesity?

In the the simplest terms, obesity occurs when energy input-calories taken in- are higher than calories expended through basal metabolic activity and exercise. Your basal metabolic rate includes the calories needed for your organ function at rest. This includes the calories needed for your heart to beat, your lungs to expand, your digestion to work and your brain to function. Exercise increases calories burned throughout the day. It increases metabolic rate and allows your metabolic rate to remain high past the time that you exercise. Your metabolic rate may be high for as long as 24 hours after exercise. Finally, exercise mobilizes white fat(storage fat) and turns it into brown fat(fat that can be burned).[1] Brown fat burns a much higher number of calories than white fat. Children have more brown fat than adults. Brown fat increases during puberty.[2] This brown fat burns more calories and keeps children's body temperature higher than adults. Lean children have more brown fat that overweight children. Inactivity and a poor diet presumable contribute to this. Exercise is the way to restore brown fat in overweight children. Puberty is a great time to establish regular exercise as it coincides with brown fat formation. We often say that children lose baby fat as teenagers. In reality, they are forming brown fat which burns more calories. No wonder they eat all the time....

How does exercise reduce the risk of type 2 diabetes?

Glucose is the fuel that is used by the body for all kinds of functions. Insulin, produced by the pancreas, keeps glucose levels in a normal range. As children become overweight, it takes higher levels of insulin to maintain a normal blood sugar. When the body can no longer keep up and insulin levels are high but not high enough to normalize blood sugar, diabetes develops. Two things happen in an overweight child. They have higher insulin levels, but their bodies are not as sensitive to the effects of insulin as their normal weight counterparts. This is called insulin resistance. Insulin resistance precedes diabetes. When you exercise, your muscles need fuel. Muscle take up glucose, reducing insulin levels and increasing the sensitivity of your body to circulating insulin.[3] This is true in children as well as adults.

How does exercise improve cognitive function?

Physical exercise increases blood flow to the brain. Children who are physically fit have measurably larger hippocampi and basal ganglia.[4] These are areas of the brain that are involved with complex memory function , attention and behavior. Children who are fit perform measurably better when given complex tasks. In a study from Health Psychology, children who were overweight and began a regular fitness program, performed higher on cognitive tasks at the conclusion of the study. The more exercise they did, the more improvement there was on cognitive function.[5]

How does exercise improve bone strength?

Bones are an active organ, constantly both forming and breaking down. Childhood and adolescence are a time of high bone growth. Peak bone mass is achieved around age 30 and declines following that. Weight bearing exercise in childhood, both aerobic and resistance exercise, causes bones to get stronger.[6] This protects children against fractures. Whether the benefit carries through to adulthood is unclear. More likely, lifelong exercise is necessary to maximizing and maintaining bone strength.

How does exercise improve mood?

Research in adults has shown that exercise increases release of endorphins. These chemicals act on the brain, causing a decrease in the perception of pain and a sedative effect. Endorphins also reduce stress and anxiety and create a feeling of positive energy. A study in 9-10 year old children confirms that children also get these same benefits from exercise.[7]

How does exercise improve sleep?

Regular, aerobic exercise reduces sleep latency, the time it takes to fall asleep, as well as improves sleep quality in children.[8] Sleep quality is better because you achieve longer periods of deep sleep. Deep sleep is restorative to the body. We know that exercise increases body temperature. Following that, body temperature declines and may make it easier to fall and stay asleep. Exercise right before bed interferes with sleep because your body temperature is still high.

What effect does resistance exercise have on children?

Past thinking held that resistance exercise was too difficult and potentially harmful for children. The picture of a child straining to lift heavy weights is not a good one.

Children are growing and their joints and tendons are not as strong as their adult counterparts. It is natural to worry about injuring children with resistance training. There is emerging research on this subject. The results are surprising. When children do resistance training, their muscles don't get bulky but they do get long and lean. They get stronger, but the strength they build seems to come from changes in nerve pathways to the brain, rather than from building big muscles.[9] They lay down communication pathways from the brain to the muscles. The brain in children 7-12 is especially receptive to strength training because their neural pathways are more "plastic" or malleable than in adolescents or adults. This is the perfect time for children to begin resistance training. The Council on Sports Medicine and Fitness has published an extensive review of strength training for children and adolescents which is an excellent resource for parents.[10]

CHAPTER FOUR
THE FITKIDS PROGRAM

by Brandon McIntosh

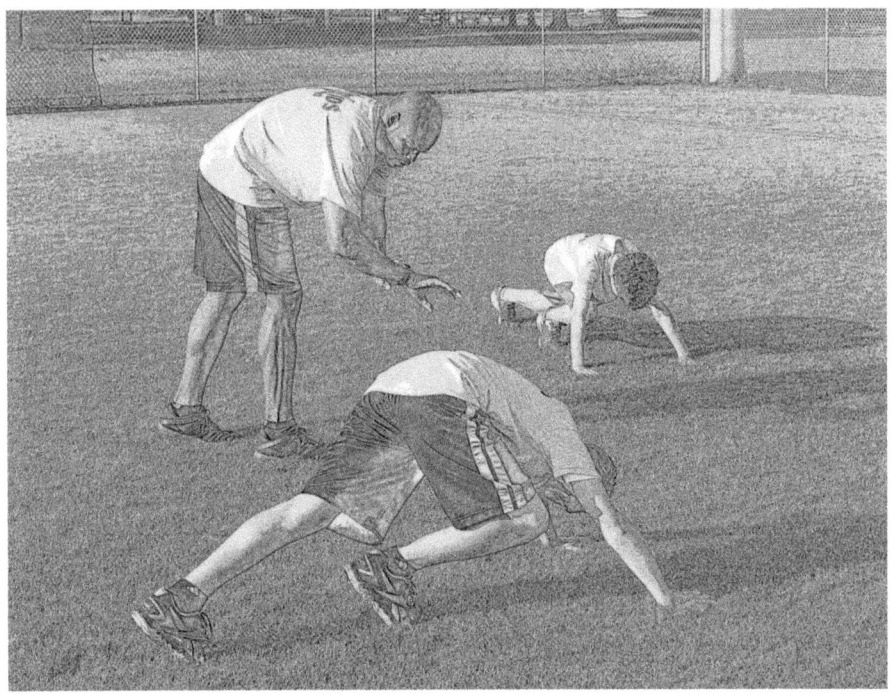

FITKIDS at Southwest Recreation Center began in May 2010. The last two years have been an incredible experience for me. I could see the change in children as they got fit and strong. They built not only physical strength but emotional strength. This program is my baby and the kids' path to a healthy future.

THE MISSION

To create a comprehensive program of exercise and nutrition for children 6-15 in a group environment. The exercises are strenuous and challenging. The nutrition portion includes education and accountablility through food logs. Motivation comes from being in a respectful, fun environment where children are positively reinforced by me, the coach and by each other. There is a constant flow of new ideas and exercises to match the energy of children.

THE METHODS

- ⚔ Creating new exercises that constantly challenge the kids, without exposing them to injury.
- ⚔ Providing individual attention to each child and addressing their needs.
- ⚔ Building an environment of striving that is positively reinforced.
- ⚔ Doing monthly challenge tests. This may track the number of push ups, sit ups, squats   or pull-ups the kids can do. Seeing their progress is a strong motivating force for them.
- ⚔ Reviewing food logs and discussing improvements than can be made.
- ⚔ Food challenges ie. A month without fast food.
- ⚔ Rewarding the child with the best food log on occasion.
- ⚔ Giving kids a turn at "Coach for a day". They all love being in charge.
- ⚔ Encouraging and tracking independent activity outside of this program.
- ⚔ Logging sleep time.

THE EXERCISES

I have developed a set of exercises after working with kids for two years and watching their ability and reactions. This form of training is great for children who don't do any other sports, but is also great for enhancing kids' athletic performance and building resistance to injury. Kids develop improved coordination, power, speed, and agility.

Before doing any physical activity, we stretch for five minutes. We also end each class with five minutes of stretching. It's very important to warm up and cool down. Stretching helps with flexibility and preventing injuries. Injury prevention is a major focus of the program.

Some kids hate stretching because they lack flexibility and find it boring. To make it fun, I usually sing, make funny faces, or walk around making small talk. Sometimes, I make it a competition (i.e., who can hold their toes the longest?). Competition is natural for children.

RESISTANCE EXERCISE

There are three types of training: strength, resistance, and power training. Power training is not recommended for children. Strength training is safe under supervision. It has lots of benefits for children. At first when I used free weights, I found that kids were intimidated. When I asked why, they said that working with weights seemed hard and painful. The bodybuilders they saw on television were huge. They couldn't relate to them. When the kids actually started using free weights, they often struggled and lost all proper form. I learned to focus on low weight at high repetitions, which helped to maintain proper form. Using free weights is only a small part of our routine.

In my program, we use resistance bands and the kids love it. Resistance bands are easy to use. Kids don't strain or struggle as much with weights, and they can control the movement. Better control means less chance of injury.

Most of the resistance exercises we do involve using body weight as the resistance.

Push ups, pull ups and squats are good examples.

AEROBIC EXERCISE

Going outdoors is a big part of FITKIDS. We spend lots of time in the park, running sprints, doing relay races, jumping hurdles, and doing any kind of exercise I can think of. Finally, we swim laps and use kickboards in the pool. Kids love being outdoors.

The next several pages will give you an idea of the variety of exercises I do with the kids. It is a small example of what we do. I mix it up. Each child is unique. Some kids are good at one exercise but not another. I always have a beginner and also an advanced exercise. If the exercises are too hard, kids get frustrated and want to quit. I start with exercises everyone can do. The kids who have not exercised get stronger and faster and they build confidence that they can do more.

Body Squats
Targeted Muscles: Hamstrings, Quadriceps, Calves, Abs

Benefits:
- Squats have been shown to improve the communication between your brain and your body's major muscle groups, and improve muscle memory.
- Improves balance and stability
- Strengthens the quads, glutes, and hamstrings
- Improves flexibility
- Increases speed and vertical jumps

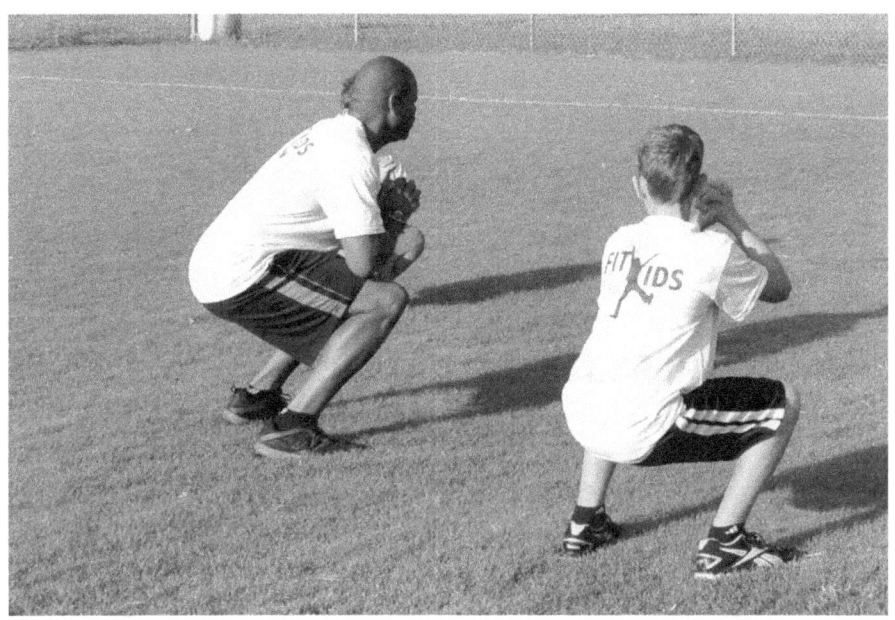

Jumping Rope
Targeted Muscles: Calves, Abs, Shoulders, Heart

Benefits:
- Burns calories
- Improves agility and speed
- Strengthens calves
- Increases aerobic capacity
- Increases stamina and endurance

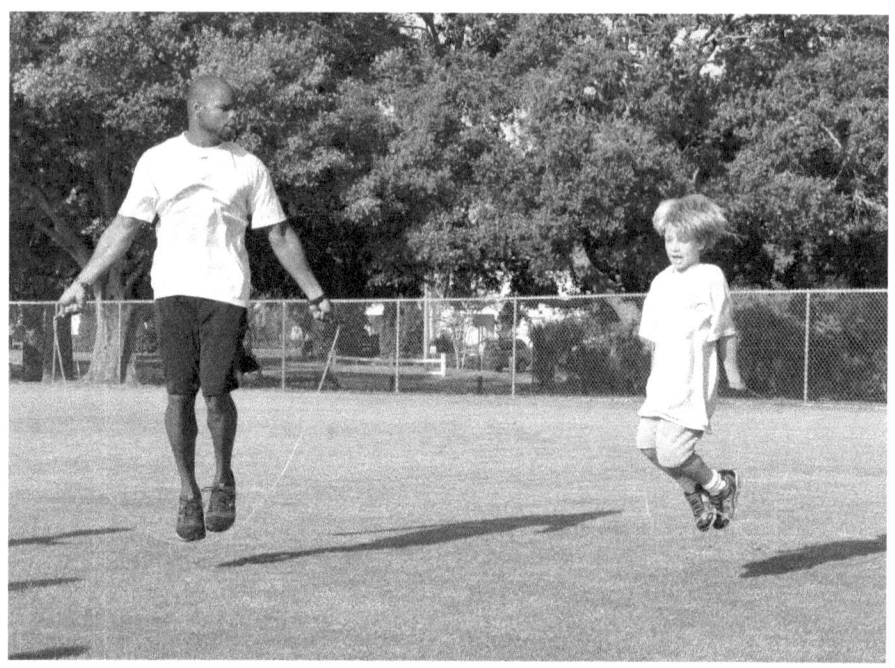

Elastic Band Biceps Curls
Targeted Muscles: Biceps

Benefits:
- ⅄ Easy free movement
- ⅄ Increases muscle strength
- ⅄ Prevent injuries

Walking Lunges
Targeted Muscles: Glutes, Hips Flexors, Quadriceps, Hamstrings

Benefits:
- ⅄ Shapes, strengthens, and tones your lower body
- ⅄ Improves speed and creates more hip flexibility
- ⅄ Helps with balance and stability

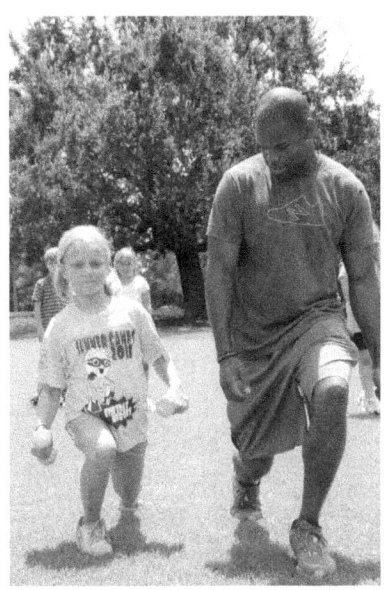

Speed Ladder Drills
Targeted Muscles: Hamstrings, Quadriceps, Calves, Hips,

Benefits:
- Improves stamina and coordination
- Increases efficiency of performance, speed, and balance
- Maintains core strength and flexibility
- Improves agility

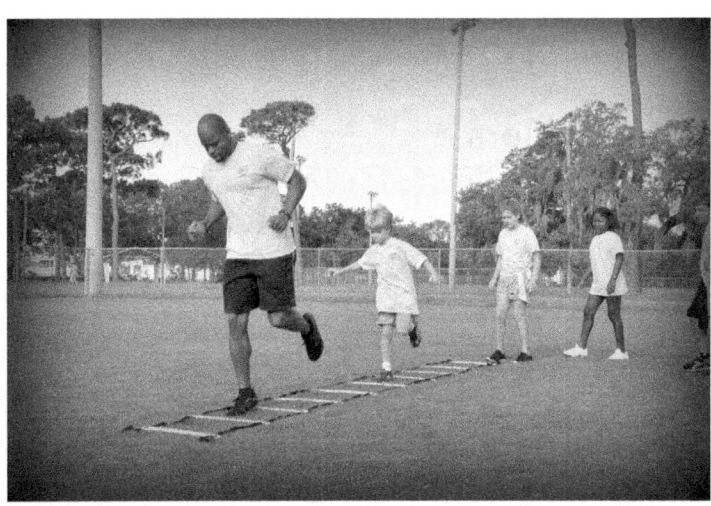

Push-ups
Targeted Muscles: Chest, Biceps, Triceps, Forearms, Shoulders, Upper Back, Glutes, Abs, Hamstrings, Quadriceps, Calves

Benefits:
- Builds strong, lean muscles
- Helps improve bone strength
- Increases heart muscle strength
- Great everyday workout!

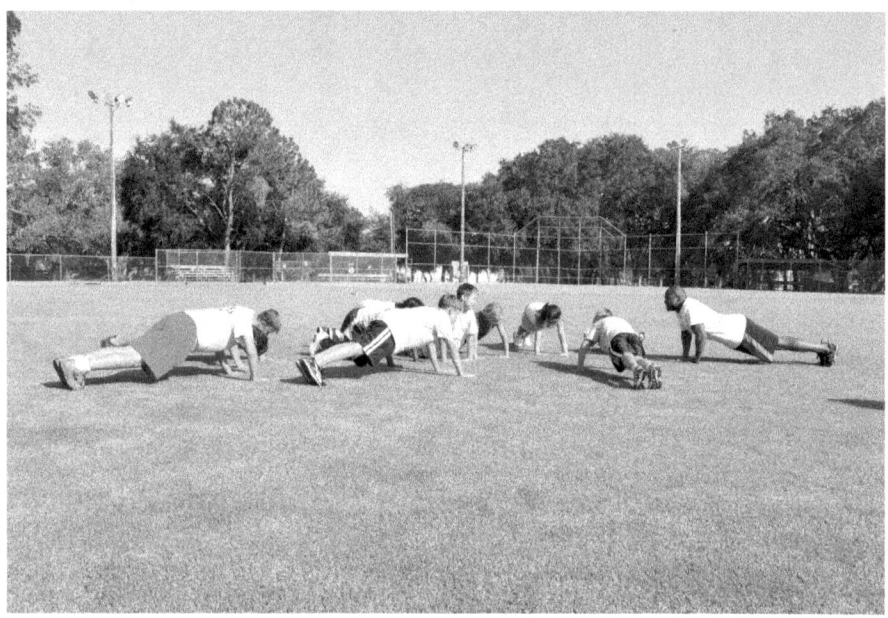

Mountain Climbers
Targeted Muscles: Glutes, Quadriceps, Rectus, Hip abductors, Hamstrings

Benefits:
- Mountain climbers are an excellent for building cardio endurance while also building core strength and agility.
- Increase endurance and stamina
- Great full body workout

Bear Crawls

Targeted Muscles: All Muscles (upper and lower body)

Benefits:
- Burns calories
- Improves coordination, agility, and speed
- Increases stamina and endurance
- Great total body workout!

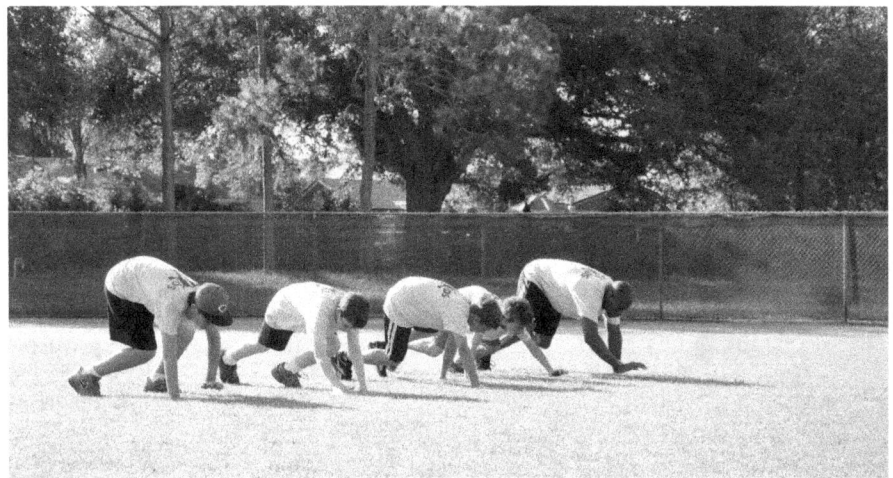

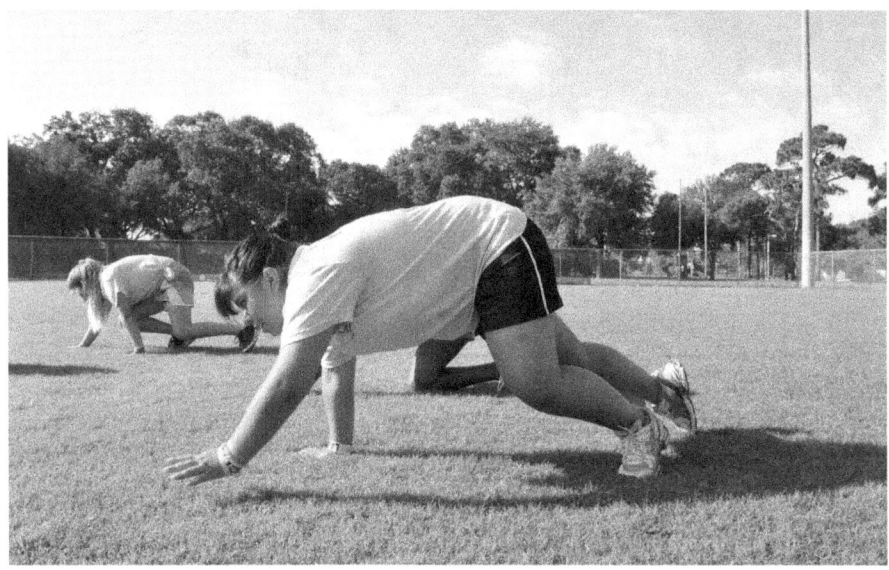

Forty-Yard Sprints
Targeted Muscles: Total Body

Benefits:
- ⅄ Burns fat and calories
- ⅄ Improves agility and speed
- ⅄ Strengthens leg muscles
- ⅄ Increases stamina and endurance
- ⅄ Kids love it!

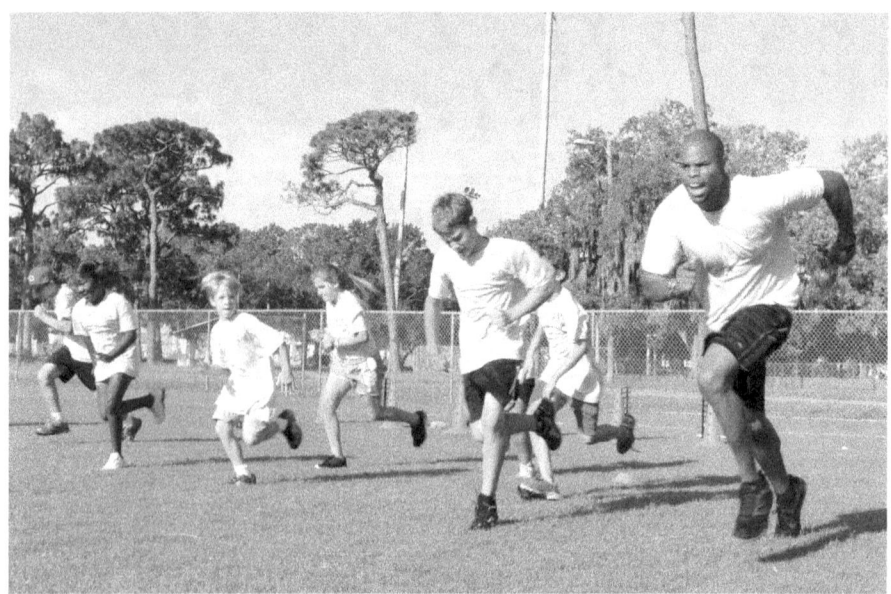

Jumping and Running Hurdles
Targeted Muscles: Hamstrings, Quadriceps, Calves, Glutes

Benefits:
- ⅄ Increases speed
- ⅄ Improves coordination
- ⅄ Strengthens calves
- ⅄ Increases stamina and endurance
- ⅄ Challenges the mind/muscle connection!

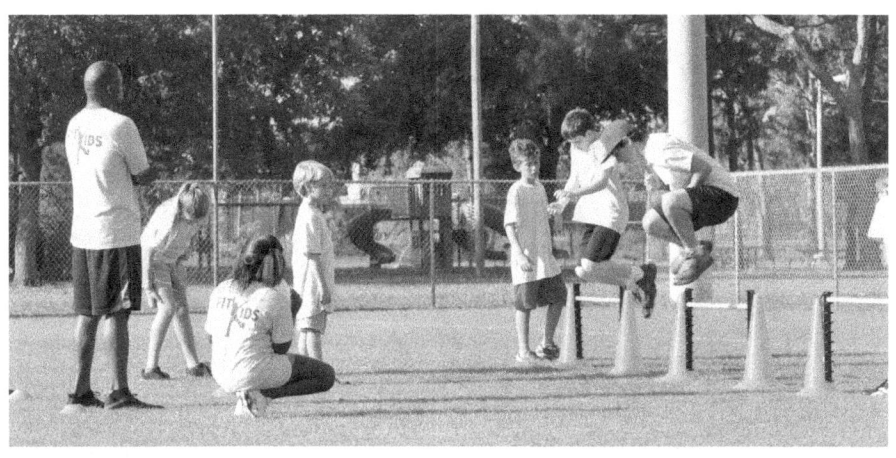

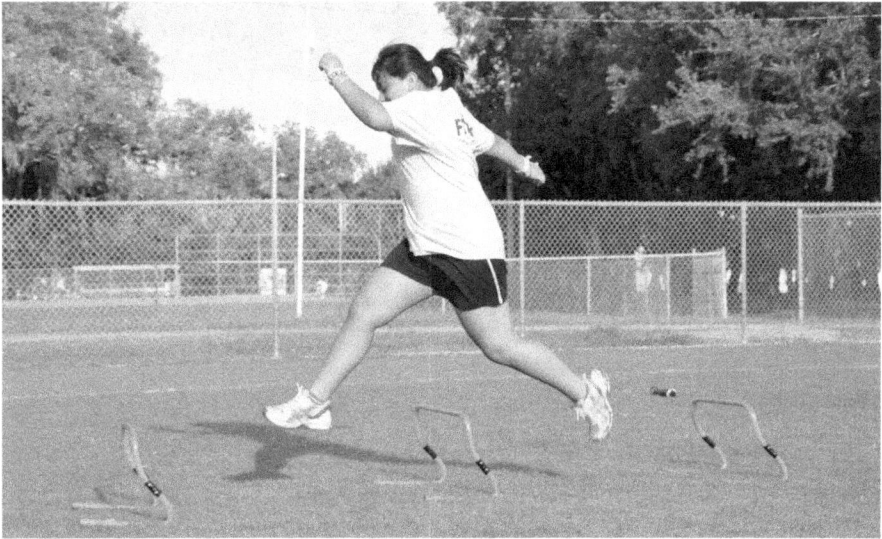

Rock Stars
Targeted Muscles: Hamstrings, Quadriceps, Calves, Glutes

Benefits:
- ⅄ *Improves* stamina and coordination
- ⅄ Increases efficiency of performance and speed
- ⅄ Helps with balance and stability
- ⅄ Strengthens the quads, glutes, and hamstrings
- ⅄ Protects against injury

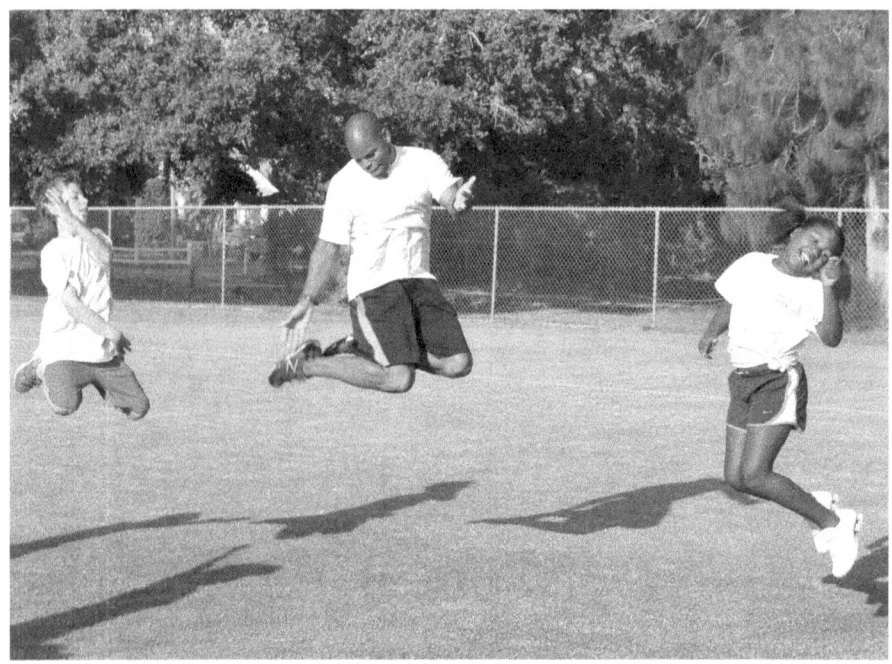

Pulling the Cattle

Targeted Muscles: All Muscles (upper and lower body)

Benefits:

- ⅄ Increases efficiency of performance and speed
- ⅄ Helps with balance and stability
- ⅄ Increases endurance and muscle strengthening
- ⅄ Burns calories
- ⅄ Protects against injury

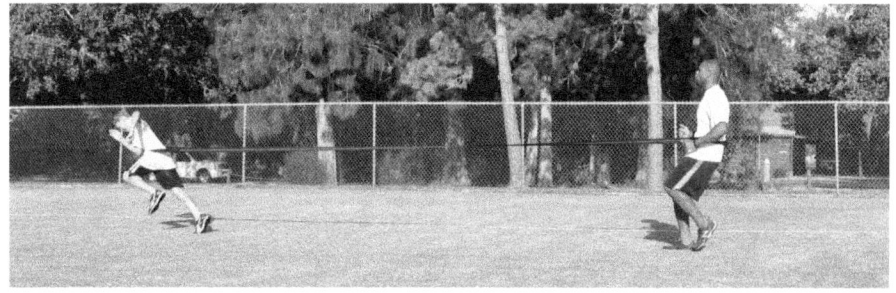

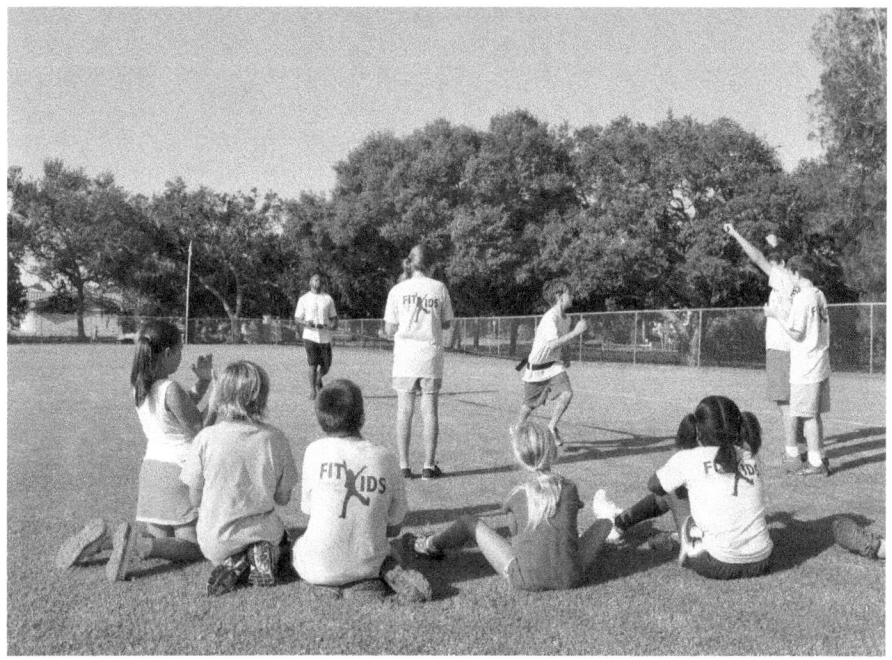

CHAPTER FIVE
THE MYSTERY OF MOTIVATION

by Chrisoula Kiriazis, MD

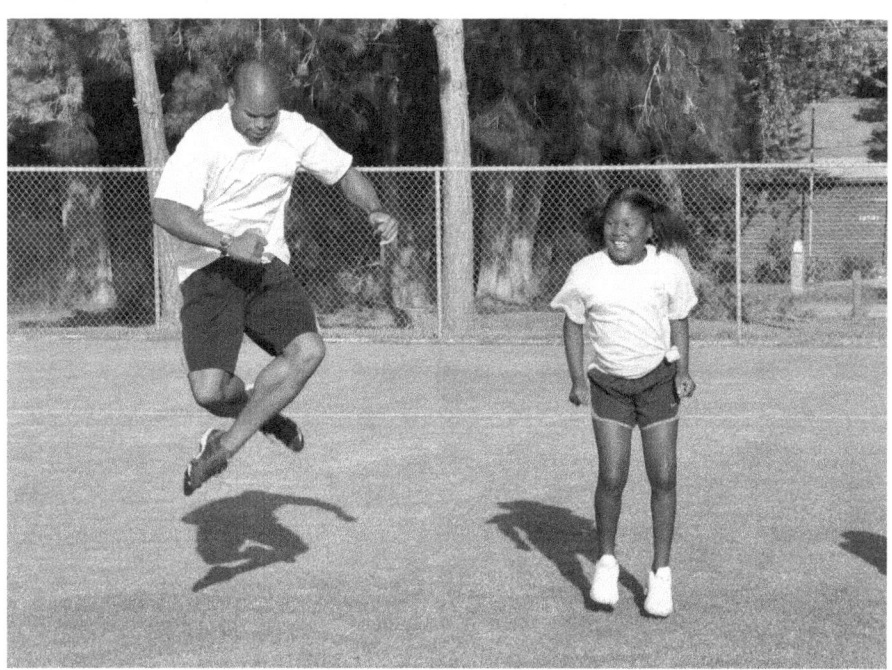

MOTIVATING PARENTS

As a doctor of many parents, there is one thing I'm very sure about: parents want what's best for their children. Their desire to help their children is very strong.

They will often change their behavior more easily if it's for their children. There is no doubt that there are obstacles— life is hectic, time is limited, money may be tight, it may be hard to change eating habits that have been part of the family for many years. All of that is true. At the same time, on a typical day, we all wake up in the morning, we all need to eat, take care of our children, and take care of all kinds of tasks, including our work, before going to sleep and doing it all over again. There are all kinds of ways that families work. Maybe parents work opposite shifts so that they don't need child care, maybe Dad is the stay-at-home parent, maybe grandparents are the caregivers while both parents work. Whichever way your family works, we all get the same amount of time to raise children—about twenty years, sometimes eighteen and sometimes twenty-five or more. In that time, we want to see our children grow into healthy, happy, productive human beings. We want those years to give them a good start in life. Parents, this book is meant to give you the tools to help your children succeed at being healthy. If you do that, you will also be healthier because health is contagious.

MOTIVATING CHILDREN

Sometimes it seems that parents and children speak a different language. Children may not always seem receptive to ideas that parents come up with. Trying to force children to do an activity they aren't interested in doesn't work very well. For the parent, trying to be an enforcer isn't much fun either. The challenge is to find the key that motivates your child. How do we motivate children to be physically active? Here are some ideas.

1. Be a good role model. Adopt a regular exercise routine. It can be as simple as walking.
2. Spend time being active together. Throw a ball, ride a bike, take a walk, hike a trail, swim, play tennis or ping pong…the choices are endless. The younger your child, the less exercise you will get, but like with providing a healthy diet, you are building the foundation of a lifelong athlete.

3. Let your child try different sports and activities, especially those that friends are participating in.
4. Educate children about the importance and benefits of exercise.
5. Enforce screen time limits. The average American child gets more than six hours of screen time daily. Why is that?
6. When children do play video games, make sure that some of them are active.
7. Take televisions and computers out of the bedroom.
8. Encourage children to go outdoors. If your neighborhood isn't appropriate, find a local park.
9. Barter screen time for exercise/outdoor time. After two hours of screen time, it's time for one hour of activity.
10. Create goals that involve training for an activity. A local five-mile walk/run is a great way to motivate the whole family to improve their level of fitness.

The magic of motivation in FITKIDS is having a coach who is interested in helping every child and in teaching them the value of working hard at exercise. The idea of striving is very important to imbed in the heart and soul of children.

Children are very capable of achieving all sorts of things if we present them with the tools they need.

Brandon is definitely a "kid whisperer." He encourages children to put forward their best effort in everything they do and rewards them with lots of praise when they achieve their goals. The mission of FITKIDS is to educate and motivate children to be healthy by having them participate in physical activity that is challenging and fun and also to make them understand the effect that their diet has on their health. Hopefully, they will become lifelong active adults.

CHAPTER SIX
MY MOTIVATION

by Brandon McIntosh

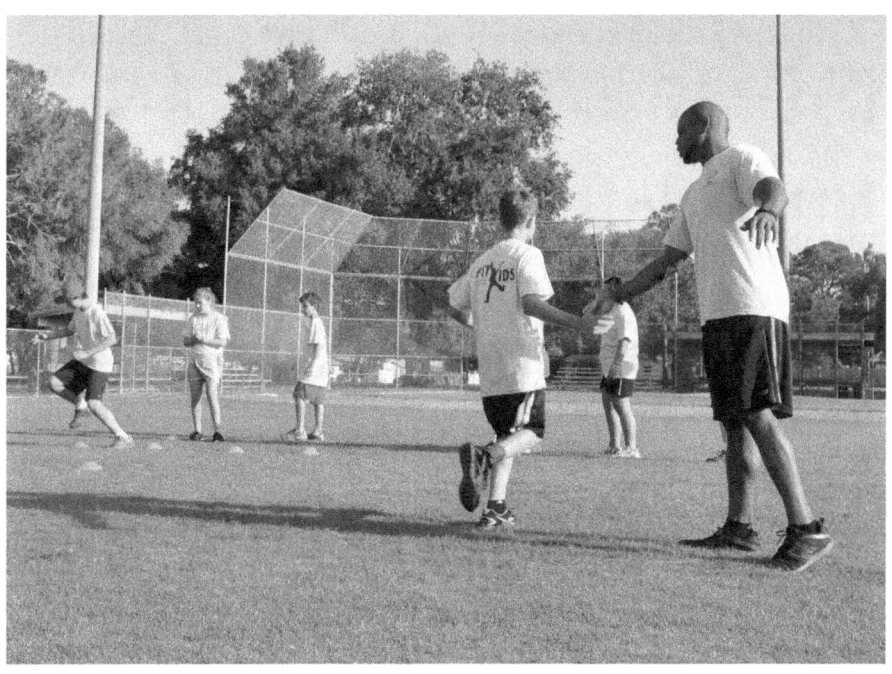

My motivation comes from my childhood. I played football growing up. I was always told that I was too short and not big enough to play. But I kept my feet moving and I never gave up. The result: a partial scholarship to college, where I played football. No one can tell you what you can't do but you!! I've had a lot of tough obstacles cross my path, both in sports and in life. Great athletes have inspired and uplifted me during difficult times. Satchel Paige said, "Never let your head hang down. Never give up and sit down and grieve. Find another way." One of my college coaches always used this quote from Ed Macauley: "When you are not training, someone somewhere is training, and when you meet him, he will win."

My main goal now is to motivate, inspire, and help children achieve their goals. Nothing motivates me more than to see a kid who wants to be the best that he or she can be.

I tell my kids every day, "If you don't give one hundred percent, you are not hurting anyone but yourself." At the same time, as Vince Lombardi said, "The strength of the group is the strength of the leaders." I love this quote because if I'm not a good leader for my kids, how can I expect them to succeed? If I'm not knowledgeable, positive, or leading by example, I would be doing a terrible job. I see it all the time in youth sports. Coaches who are overweight tell their players to eat better and stay in shape. They come to the field with fast food and can't run a lap. That's how you lose respect from your players or the kids you train.

What I have seen is that kids motivate each other. Being in a group, rather than one-on-one personal training, creates a team environment that helps to encourage kids to try harder at whatever exercise they are doing. I learned to be careful and treat each child as an individual. The kids come from different backgrounds, in different sizes, with different personalities. I demand that they respect each other. Next, I have to find challenging exercises that are not too overwhelming and can be done at different levels.

Kids who are just starting do fewer repetitions of any exercise. As kids improve, they are willing and able to do more.

Food logs are a great motivating force in FITKIDS. Writing down what kids eat gives them the chance to think about what they're eating. Just having to write it down makes it likelier that kids will eat healthy foods. Next, I review food logs and talk about what improvements can be made. Sometimes, I make it a competition and reward the person who has eaten the best over the last week. This is where I need the help of parents. Kids can make better choices if they have healthy food at home. The success of eating better begins with the person who does the shopping. My next goal is to incorporate nutritional consultation with each family who participates in FITKIDS.

CHAPTER SEVEN
A WORD FROM THE KIDS

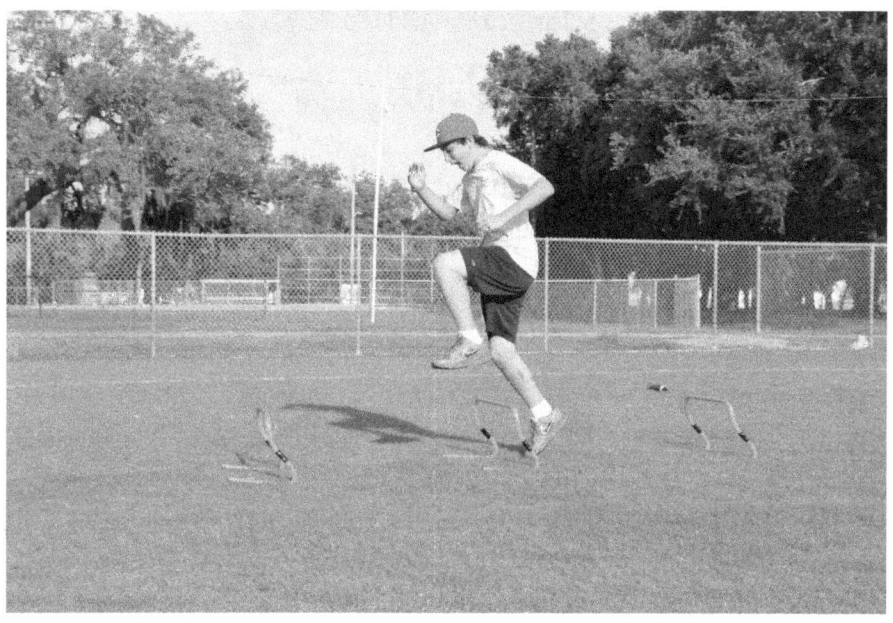

Noah Aktas
Age 12
First day at Fit Kids: May 9th, 2010(His Birthday)

When I first started Fit Kids, I always said to myself stuff like, "I'm fat, I can't do it, it's too hard." I was approximately 140 pounds when I started to lose weight. Before I knew it, I was 130 pounds and working out was easy. Now, I'm 118 pounds and the workouts Brandon makes me do are so easy. Brandon is more than just a fitness instructor, he's basically family. I have known him for so long. If it weren't for him, I would be sitting on a couch eating chips and watching television. Because of him, now I play two sports going on three. I work out with him every Monday and Thursday and play football on Saturday. If you know Brandon, then you're very lucky.

Winchester Dermody
Age 12
First day at Fit Kids: June 7th, 2010

Fit Kids has helped me increase my confidence when participating in physical activities and helped me become stronger. I know Coach Brandon has our best interests in mind.

He has made us stronger in so many ways, not just physically. I could work out at home, but when I go to Fit Kids, we do something new each day. The variety is what makes Fit Kids fun. It's not just exercising; it's challenging each other with new workouts and competing with your friends. Once I joined, I knew that within the program, we didn't just push ourselves, we pushed each other.

I have learned that if you don't eat properly, it doesn't matter if you exercise or not, so some days we take nutrition lessons with Coach Brandon. Fit Kids has helped boost my health. I was always fit, but Fit Kids increased my hand eye coordination, made me stronger, made me faster, and increased my endurance. You don't just become fit, you become superfit. Coach Brandon has helped me in so many ways, to the point where I don't think of Brandon as my coach any more, I think of him as my friend as well.

Zachary Dermody
Age 10
First Day at Fit Kids: June 7, 2010

When I first started Fit kids, I wasn't as fast. Fit kids pushed me to the limit. It improved my stamina. It improved more than just my speed. It made me a much stronger person too. I can do a pull up. Fit kids works your core which really helps with sit ups. I am a very good jumper and Fit Kids has challenged me. I can run as fast a cheetah. I am as strong as an ox, and I can jump as far as a kangaroo.

It has also been a very fun experience.

It has also helped me in other situations, from school to sports. For example, when I don't think I can do something, I just think that I've pushed myself before so I can do it again.

CHAPTER EIGHT
FOOD FOR THOUGHT: TWELVE RULES FOR BETTER NUTRITION

by Chrisoula Kiriazis, MD

1. Always make sure that you and your children eat breakfast. Avoid high-sugar cereals. Do add protein in the form of milk, yogurt, eggs, or nuts.
2. Limit the amount of white stuff in your diet—less white rice, white potatoes, white pasta, white bread, and sugar, including high-fructose corn syrup. In contrast, whole grains are a great fuel for active children. They provide fiber, nutrients, and energy.
3. Eat fish at least once or twice per week. Canned chunk light tuna and canned sardines are easy and good for you.
4. Eat less saturated fat. Limit red meat to once per week, use small amounts of butter, whole milk, and cheese in your diet, and stop frying food.
5. Eat lots of fresh fruit and vegetables on a daily basis. Wash all of it and peel some of it. Steam or microwave vegetables that need to be cooked. Avoid cooked carrots, creamed corn, and peas, which are very high in sugar. Canned fruit is not a fruit but a dessert full of sugar.

6. Help your children to make their own lunch for school. Leftovers are a great choice. Don't add sugary snacks to their lunch. They will usually eat the snacks first and throw away the rest. Fruit or raw carrots are a great addition for lunch.

7. Stop drinking soda and fruit juice (with the exception of orange juice). Really! Drink milk or calcium-enriched soy milk or orange juice to give growing bones what they need.

8. READ FOOD LABELS and avoid foods with TRANS FAT. That means margarine and many types of cookies and crackers.

9. Graze—eating small, frequent meals—to keep your metabolism going. Remember that grazing involves chewing slowly. Fruit and nuts are a great snack.

10. Make friends with your kitchen and local produce market and drag your children along for the ride occasionally. Shopping and cooking are much more fun when you're not doing it alone. Commit to trying new foods. Have your children assist with meal preparation.

11. Try to have dinner together as a family. Make one meal for everyone and turn off the television.

12. Get your ZZZs. Children need nine to eleven hours of sleep each night. A quiet, dark place without a television, cell phone, or computer nearby is best.

CHAPTER NINE
THE CHALLENGE FOR PARENTS

Good nutrition is a building block for good health throughout life. Nutrition for children begins in the womb. Mom, being at a healthy weight, exercising during pregnancy, eating a healthy diet and not gaining excessive weight during pregnancy will be beneficial to you and your baby. Breastfeeding is healthier than bottle feeding and reduces your child's chance of being overweight.

Even though I am a doctor, it has been a journey to become knowledgeable about nutrition and, more importantly, to put that knowledge into practice, day after day, meal after meal. Becoming a parent has put my commitment to a healthy lifestyle to the test.

As a parent working full-time with two boys, now aged ten and twelve, preparing healthy food takes some planning. I think that most of us have a passion for eating. The next step is to make that a passion for eating well. When you are a parent, eating well and teaching your children to eat well brings you huge rewards.

First, you have to shop for food. To all those parents navigating the grocery store with one or more toddler, my hat is off to you. The choices of packaged, prepared, and instant foods are amazing and endless. To the sleep-deprived, harried parent trying to get out of the store, the draw of these meals is very powerful. What could be more wonderful than microwave pizza at the end of a long day at work? Kraft Mac and Cheese, of course!

Next, you have to prepare meals. While it may seem like a time-consuming task, cooking a simple meal can take as little as thirty minutes. Short of drive-through fast food, I don't know of any restaurant that can serve a meal in less time. There are countless thirty-minute recipes out there. My favorites come from *Cooking Light*, which is my go-to resource for weeknight meals. To all those people who hate to cook, I have one piece of advice: get over it or find a partner who loves to cook. Either approach works well. For me, cooking is a creative process. The worst that can happen is you make a bad meal. The best that happens is that you make a tantalizing meal that stimulates every taste bud in your body and leaves you with a Zen-like glow of enchantment. How bad can that be?

Modeling good eating habits is important for you as a parent. You can't tell your child to eat raw carrots while you are eating french fries and doughnuts. You need to walk the walk if you want your words to have any credibility. Actions are stronger than words. At the same time, children don't always seem to listen to their parents. Putting them in a program like FITKIDS is an incredible way to help them achieve lifelong good habits and to learn more yourself. The message will be coming from someone who is not a parent but who they respect and are willing to learn from. We all know that children sometimes seem to have better hearing when it's not Mom and Dad talking. Finally, the goal of FITKIDS is to encourage discussion about nutrition, hopefully at the dinner table, while you are enjoying a good meal together.

CHAPTER TEN
CHILDREN AND THEIR EATING
LANDSCAPE

Children definitely alter the eating landscape. First, the adorable but incredibly demanding little people have to be fed one spoonful at a time. It all starts out with mush and then moves on to ground-up or carefully cut-up chunks of food, some of which inevitably lodge in their throats while they are carefully strapped into a high chair. Fortunately, children keep eating new and bigger things all the time. The going can be quite slow. Chewing raw carrots while losing baby teeth doesn't work well. I don't think salad became part of our dinner meal until the kids were over five. By the time they were five, we were ready to explore all kinds of new foods. I say "we" meaning my husband and I. My children were not culinary adventurers. Having to eat crab cakes and vegetable lasagna reduced them to tears for the pure torture of it.

We know that children's taste buds are still developing. They like sweet flavors and dislike bitter ones. Over time, that changes. Refusing to eat new foods beyond a certain age becomes a behavioral trait. Parents, if you have given up after fighting the good fight, I am here to remind you that there is life beyond mac and cheese, pizza, and hot dogs. Make one meal for the entire family. Don't make the dinner table a battleground but do continue to introduce new foods. Engage your children in this process. Educate them. Let them know that hating mushrooms at age five does not destine them to a life without portabellas.

Children can be very good at regulating their food intake. Forcing them to "clean their plate" takes away their innate ability to stop eating when they are not hungry and may lead to adult obesity. Serve small portions. Encourage them to eat slowly and stop before they are stuffed. We have met children who have bragged about the number of slices of pizza they could eat. Eating large quantities of food is not desirable but it is a very common bad habit.

CHAPTER ELEVEN
RAW FOOD VS
PROCESSED FOOD

RAW FOOD

Let's talk about raw food. Raw fruit and vegetables, with rare exceptions, offer the highest quantities of nutrients and antioxidants. Cooked tomatoes are an exception due to higher levels of lycopene than in raw tomatoes. Your body also has to work harder to break down raw food, which has a high fiber content. The upside is that you burn more calories digesting the food. So while the calories in one cup of raw carrots is the same as in cooked carrots, the fiber in cooked carrots is broken down by the cooking process.

Your body does less work breaking down and absorbing cooked carrots so the the net calories are higher. So you see, all calories are not created equal.

Fresh fruit needs to be washed, and sometimes peeled and chopped. Unfortunately, children are not proficient with a knife until they are older, so here we go again, creating more work for the parent. Think of cutting up fruit and vegetables as depositing coins in a piggy bank. Your children will be rich in health after doing it consistently for years and you will receive the dividends related to that.

WHOLE GRAINS

Whole grains are healthy complex carbohydrates which act as a fuel for muscles.

Whole grains contain the entire seed or endosperm, germ, and bran of a grain. The body takes longer to break these down than refined grains like white rice, white bread, and white pasta, and so blood sugar does not rise as quickly or as much after eating them. Your blood sugar stays more even with whole grains. In addition, whole grains are an important source of vitamins and fiber. Examples of whole grains include: brown rice, quinoa, oats, whole grain or spelt pasta, farro, barley, whole wheat bread, and popcorn.

The more children exercise, the more they can eat. If your child sits in front of a screen for hours every day, eating lots of grains, even healthy ones, will result in being over-weight. When carbohydrates are not used to fuel muscles for exercise, they are broken down and stored as fat.

PROCESSED FOOD

On the other end of the spectrum, you definitely want to avoid processed food. What does processed food mean? Processed food is already broken down, meaning your body has to do less work to digest and absorb it. White rice con-sists of rice kernels with the husk removed. White bread is made from wheat that has been stripped of the germ and bran. What remains is a carbohydrate, which is more quickly broken down. Your intestines absorb it quickly and your blood sugar rises quickly as a result. After your blood sugar rises, insulin levels rise in response. This has the effect of bringing your blood sugar back into the normal range. Eating lots of carbohydrates can cause your insulin levels to overshoot. Three hours later, instead of your blood sugar being normal, it can get very low, which is a condition called hypoglycemia. What happens then? Usually you break into a sweat, feel that your heart is racing, and have a strong craving for food. More sugar takes away the symptoms but, three hours later, you guessed it: the same thing happens.

Eating processed food leads to a roller coaster of insulin and blood sugar levels. The larger the portions, the worse the reaction. If you are overweight and have insulin levels that are high for long periods of time, your pancreas, the gland in your body that produces insulin, can't keep up. It is like a treadmill where you fall further and further behind. Meanwhile, as you gain weight, your body becomes less sensitive to the insulin floating around in your bloodstream. The insulin is knocking on the door, asking to come in, but the doors are shut. This is the process that leads to diabetes. We never saw this kind of diabetes in children until obesity in kids became a common condition.

HIGH-FRUCTOSE CORN SYRUP AND SUGAR

High-fructose corn syrup is a processed sugar that comes from corn. Soda of all kinds, noncarbonated drinks like lemonade, and marshmallows are all examples of foods that contain high-fructose corn syrup. High-fructose corn syrup has invaded our food supply because it is cheap and easy to use. It is the basis of the soda empire of the world. It is really hard to find any redeeming qualities about soda except it tastes good. It is thirst-quenching in a way that water is not. It seems especially helpful when you are fighting a gastrointestinal bug or you feel nauseated for any reason. I think that covers the positives.

The negatives are much more compelling. In a California study, kids drinking one can of soda a day were 60 percent more likely to be overweight.[11] One soda daily amounts to 39 pounds of sugar for the year. Drinking calories does not decrease the amount of calories you consume in food. Truly, it is a lose-lose proposition. First, you consume junk calories with no nutritional value and, second, you greatly increase your chance of being obese.

There is no evidence that high-fructose corn syrup is unhealthier than plain old sugar but high-fructose corn syrup has replaced sugar to such a degree that it represents a big part of our obesity problem.

For all those parents, like my husband and me, who avoided soda, we often made different mistakes. I regularly gave my children apple juice as toddlers, thinking I was giving them something healthy. Twelve cavities later, my dentist enlightened me. Any sweet drink will lodge between teeth more effectively than cookies or cake. Considering the manual dexterity of kids and their lack of ability and enthusiasm to thoroughly brush and floss their teeth, that leads to a perfect storm of cavities. Needless to say, other than orange juice, which has a lower sugar content when it is natural, there aren't many juices in our pantry. Drinking sweetened juice has a similar effects on weight as drinking soda.[12]

Juice does provide some of the antioxidants of real fruit but lacks all the fiber content. An apple is healthier than apple juice, oranges are healthier than orange juice, grapes are healthier than grape juice, etc. Once again, taking away the fiber in fruit makes it easier for our bodies to absorb. Your sugar level goes right up after drinking juice.

CHAPTER TWELVE
GOOD FAT VS BAD FAT

GOOD FAT VS. BAD FAT

We need fat in our diets—that is why omega-3 and -6 fatty acids are called "essential."

Plants contain essential fatty acids—both omega-3 and omega-6 fatty acids—that human beings need and cannot produce for themselves. They are called "essential" because they are necessary for the normal functioning of our immune system, our kidneys, and our skin, to name just a few things. Omega-3 and omega-6 fatty acids are examples of polyunsaturated fats. While fish contain omega-3 oils, they have them because they eat plants (for example, algae) that make these. Other plants that make essential fatty acids include leafy vegetables, nuts, seeds, flax, and soybean. Tofu, which is made from soybeans, is an excellent source of omega fatty acid as well as protein. For vegetarians, who don't eat animal protein, tofu is a very important part of their diet.

Monounsaturated fat is found in olive, canola, and peanut oils, and avocados. Eating monounsaturated fats will lower your cholesterol and, with it, your risk of heart disease.

Polyunsaturated fats are found in fish and have great health benefits. Mono- and polyunsaturated fats are GOOD FATS.

Saturated fat is BAD FAT. It is found in butter, fatty meats—red meat, chicken with skin, fatty pork—and dairy products, including whole milk and cheese. These foods are high in calories and increase your cholesterol and risk of heart disease. The Atkins Diet should be called the Heart Disease Diet because it is full of saturated fat. We should be eating small amounts of saturated fat. Limit red meat intake to once a week, choose leaner cuts of meat, trim the fat before cooking meats, choose chicken without skin, don't fry foods, and use small amounts of butter in conjunction with olive or canola oil to add taste.

THE FISH STORY

Fish is an excellent example of good fat. Omega-3 fish oils , found in fish, are important for brain development—in fact, pregnant women who consume high quantities of fish have babies with measurably higher IQs. Fish oil is also important for the functioning of joints and reduces inflammation and the risk of heart disease and cancer. The fish highest in fish oil are sardines and mackerel. Salmon has intermediate levels and tuna has lower levels of fat than other fish.

There are concerns about our fish supply, however. Fish are consuming mercury, which is polluting the water. The longest-living and largest fish accumulate the most mercury. Avoid eating sharks, swordfish, king mackerel, or tilefish because of their high mercury content. Sushi lovers who eat blue fin and yellow fin tuna on a regular basis have measurably elevated mercury levels. Canned chunk light tuna contains much less mercury than either albacore or tuna served in restaurants. Children are more susceptible to the effects of mercury because it affects their developing nervous system.

Wild salmon is the healthiest type of salmon; it gets its pink color from its diet of shrimp. Farmed salmon aren't fed shrimp. They get fish meal that can be high in a chemical called PCB. Fish meal is fed to farmed salmon to give it its pretty pink color but the PCBs are harmful. PCB is a cancer-causing chemical and is felt to be dangerous to humans if consumed frequently. It is safest to limit eating farmed salmon to once a month.

The alternative now is salmon color-enhanced through feed. In color-enhanced salmon, the fish meal contains the same chemical that gives shrimp its pink color naturally. Salmon gets a pink color without a toxic chemical. However, the quality of fish meal fed to farmed salmon varies greatly and farmed salmon is lower in omega-3 fish oil than wild salmon.

The growing brains of children may be more susceptible to toxins, so choose your fish wisely.

THE EGG STORY

Eggs, used to be thought of as bad fat but the pendulum has swung back to the center. Egg yolks contain both essential fatty acids (good fat) and saturated fat (bad fat). Egg whites contain protein with very little fat or carbohydrate. Eggs are a great source of protein and vitamins, including vitamins A, D, E, and K. Up to seventy percent of people who eat eggs don't have much change in their cholesterol. Children definitely benefit from having eggs in their diet.

Cooking eggs thoroughly helps to kill any bacteria—like salmonella—that may have contaminated them. Who knew that you were taking your life in your mouth by enjoying the soft gooeyness of a soft boiled egg?

So, that's the egg story. Eggs can be part of a healthy diet for children. The things we add to them are not healthy: bacon, grits, biscuits with gravy, home fries with a side of toast slathered in butter...well, need I say more?

PARTIALLY HYDROGENATED VEGETABLE OIL

Let's talk about another manmade BAD FAT: partially hydrogenated vegetable oil (PHVO). What happens when you take regular vegetable oil—usually corn, soybean, palm, or canola—and heat it to high levels? Presto—partially hydrogenated oils are created. These are also known as trans fat. Margarine is the most common trans fat that doesn't hide in baked goods. For years, margarine was felt to be healthier than butter. This isn't true. Trans fats are as bad for your heart as the fat in butter. We know that when vegetable oils are heated to high levels, free radicals are produced. Free radicals contribute to cancer.

Why do we use trans fats then? We use them because they are excellent preservatives. Cookies made with PHVO can last for months. Convenience and longevity trumps healthy food for the big producers of food supply. Slowly, though, just like an invasion that gradually recedes, the more we talk about this issue, the more that big food producers start to pay attention and remove trans fat from food. Finding labels that say "0 Trans Fat" is now pretty common. Look for them and please don't eat margarine (good alternatives are Smart Balance and, my preference, Soy Free Earth Balance).

LOW-FAT FOODS

We have become the fattest nation in the world with the greatest number of low- and non-fat foods on our store shelves. As we discussed, not all fat is bad. Be careful, non-fat often means higher in carbohydrates with a modest reduction in calories. If you compare labels, you will see that non-fat yogurt tends to be higher in carbohydrate content, which is not necessarily better for you. Low-fat is a better choice.

The great thing about fat is its satiety value. Eating one piece of fried chicken goes a long way in making you feel full. A whole bowl of stir fried rice won't go as far in satis-fying hunger. Fat doesn't trigger insulin shifts the way that carbohydrates do, so you won't feel like eating again in two hours. The trick is to eat small amounts of fat. Getting fat from nuts, vegetables, and fish is healthier than getting fat from meat, butter, fried foods, and cheese. But really the key is moderation.

CHAPTER THIRTEEN
ADDITIVES IN FOODS

SUGAR-FREE FOODS

Sugar-free foods have also proliferated on our store shelves. Sugar free usually means that artificial sugar has been added. Examples of artificial sugar include sucralose (Splenda), sacharrin (Sweet'N Low) and aspartame(Equal). This has been a great invention for diabetics, who have to be very careful about the carbohydrates they consume. For the rest of us, I don't think sugar substitutes offer any great benefit. Both children and adults who consume diet drinks may be heavier. It is not clear exactly why that is. It may be that even though sugar substitutes are free of calories, the brain responds to them in the same way as regular sugar, setting up a craving for more sweets.

The safety of artificial sugars has been questioned, though there has been no proof that they are harmful. The newest alternative, Stevia, is natural, though that we don't have proof that it is better. Children are better off with less of these chemicals since the long term effects are not known.

HORMONES AND ANTIBIOTICS IN FOODS

Modern farming has become very successful in producing large quantities of food quickly. Unfortunately, some of their practices are definitely questionable, if not outright harmful. Hormones added to animal feed help animals to grow faster.

What happens when our children consume chicken, pork, beef, eggs, and milk full of hormones? We don't know. We do know that puberty is starting awfully early these days and there is concern that hormones derived from foods may contribute. Think about it: we have made androgenic steroids illegal but allow hormones in our food supply. What about antibiotics used in feed to prevent infection, illness, and death in animals? There is a rising tide of bacteria resistant to the antibiotics we use to combat disease. The factors contributing to this include overuse of antibiotics to treat illnesses like colds and bronchitis and also possibly the use of antibiotics in farming.

Antibiotic use may not seem very concerning to you but it should be. New information is showing that the use of antibiotics alters the makeup of bacteria in the stomach and gastrointestinal system. Bacteria normally live throughout the gastrointestinal tract, which starts in your mouth and goes to the esophagus, stomach, small, and finally large intestine. The kinds of bacteria that live in your body help to determine how food is broken down when it begins its trek from your mouth to the outside world. Some bacteria are much more efficient at breaking down food and extracting every last calorie from the food you eat. Taking antibiotics makes your gut flora—the bacteria in your gut—change for up to one year, and that has an effect on how your food is digested and absorbed. Do you want to give your children foods that contain antibiotics if this increases their risk of being overweight?

CHEMICALS AND PESTICIDES IN FOODS

We may not have all the information, but consumers are concerned enough about chemicals and pesticides in foods that organic and natural foods are everywhere.

Organic and natural are not the same. Organic foods mean that the food is produced, manufactured, and handled using organic means—that means free of chemical fertilizers, pesticides, and preservatives. Organic foods are monitored and regulated by the US Department of Agriculture. Natural foods mean that the food is derived from plants and animals rather than being manufactured, like Velveeta cheese, for example.

We don't have any proof that organic foods are healthier but we do have some proof that pesticides and chemicals used to grow foods are harmful to humans. There is a debate about how much is harmful. The current levels of pesticides that are used in making our food adhere to old guidelines that experts feel are too liberal. While washing and peeling fruit helps remove pesticides, cooking does not reliably remove chemicals from some foods. Here is a list of foods that are high in pesticides. They are called the "Dirty Dozen": 1. apples 2. celery 3. strawberries 4. peaches 5. spinach 6. nectarines 7. imported grapes 8. sweet bell peppers 9. potatoes 10. blueberries 11. lettuce 12. kale. Eating smaller quantities of these foods or choosing organic versions is recommended.

While everyone agrees that it is healthier to eat fruit and vegetables because of the nutrients they contain, the pesticides are also there. Americans use more than a billion pounds of pesticides each year. Children are more susceptible to the effects of these chemicals because they are still developing. Toxicity to children from pesticides affects their nervous systems. Consider organic milk, and limit the amount of orange juice or applesauce your children are consuming.

There is a reason that chemicals and pesticides are added to our foods: bacteria do contaminate our food supply. The Center for Disease Control estimates that food-borne illness, usually caused by bacteria contaminating our foods, takes an annual toll of three thousand deaths per year. Peanut butter, tomatoes, alfalfa, spinach, and ground beef are all examples of foods containing bacteria that have led to epidemics of illness in the United States in the last few years. What can you do as a parent? Wash and rinse all foods, peel or avoid fruit high in pesticides, and cook all ground meat, poultry roasts and pork to medium well done to destroy any bacteria. Steaks and chicken breasts need to be completely seared on the outside, without being cut open during cooking. Be careful about foods that have not been refrigerated for hours, like picnic and buffet food.

NITRITES AND NITRATES IN FOODS

Nitrites are salts used to cure meats including deli meat, bacon and hot dogs.

There is concern that these chemicals are harmful. They are used because they reduce the growth of bacteria and help prevent botulism in our foods. Nitrites can, under certain circumstances, develop into nitrosamines which are carcinogenic. Vitamin C reduces this risk.

Eighty percent of the nitrites in our body come from vegetables grown in nitrogen rich soil(which is provided by fertilizers). Vegetables contain nitrates rather than nitrites but our digestive system transforms them into nitrites. The vegetables highest in nitrates are spinach, lettuce, beets, radishes, celery and cabbage. It is not clear that vegetable forms of nitrates are harmful. Infants are prone to a rare condition called methemoglobinemia and should not get large amounts of these vegetables.

Nitrosamines seem to develop in higher quantities when cured meats are heated.

When bacon and hot dogs are cooked, the level of nitrosamines are higher. The more they are cooked, the higher the levels. Bacon drippings are especially high in nitrosamine content.

Children may be more susceptible to the effects of carcinogens than adults.

Limit the amount of bacon and hot dogs in your children's diet. The concern regarding deli meats is less because the quantity of nitrites is low and these meats are not heated. Furthermore, they are supplemented with vitamin c which reduces formation of nitrosamine.

CLEAR PLASTIC CONTAINERS
The containers we store our food in are also a source for concern. When certain clear plastic containers labeled with a PC#7 are heated up, they leach a chemical called BP-a (bisphenol-A). This chemical is harmful to humans at high levels and is now being removed because of concerns about its safety. Putting PC#7 plastics in the microwave and dishwasher is a practice that needs to stop. Transfer foods to a glass Pyrex dish before heating. Liners of canned food like soups, beans, and some plastic soda containers also contain BP-a. This chemical mimics the effects of female hormones and is called a hormone disruptor. Scientists studying the effects of BP-a in canned food no longer eat canned food with liners containing BP-a.

MICROWAVE POPCORN
The liner of microwave popcorn bags releases a chemical called PFOA when heated; this chemical is known to be a carcinogen. Popcorn is healthy when you pop it in a popcorn maker. The power of consumers is that we can effect change by not buying foods that are potentially harmful. Don't buy microwave popcorn.

TEFLON-COATED COOKWARE
The same chemical released from microwave popcorn bags, PFOA, is used to bond the nonstick coating to Teflon pans.

If pans are heated over 660 degrees, which will happen if they are left dry on a hot burner for a long time or if their surface is damaged by metal cooking utensils or steel wool used to clean them, they release PFOA, which is known to be a carcinogen. If used properly, nonstick cookware should pose little risk.

CHAPTER FOURTEEN
VITAMINS AND SUPPLEMENTS

Let's talk about our love affair with vitamins and supplements. The vitamin industry has a motto: if a food is found to be nutritious, then a vitamin supplement made from that food will arrive on our shelves (to name a few: fish oil, vitamins A, B, C, D, and E, pomegranate tablets, blue-green algae, etc.). For the most part, there is no proof that supplements improve our health. Our bodies don't utilize nutrients in tablet form in the same way they utilize nutrients in food form. Sometimes, high doses of manufactured vitamins may actually be harmful, as in the case of beta carotene and vitamin E.

The American Academy of Pediatrics does not recommend that children routinely receive vitamins or supplements. The most common nutritional deficiencies in children include iron and vitamin D. Lack of iron causes anemia. Lack of Vitamin D causes a bone disease called rickets. The recommended amount of Vit D daily is 200-400IU. One glass of milk, either cow or soymilk, provide 100IU Vitamin D. If you are in shorts and a tank top, 10 minutes in the sun without sunscreen may provide up to 10,000IU of Vitamin D. The recommended amount of iron for children is 8-15mg daily. Iron is present in dried beans, dried fruit, eggs, liver and red meat, chicken, salmon, tuna, broccoli, spinach, wheat, pasta and rice. Even if your child is a picky eater, supplements found in cereal, milk and orange juice will usually prevent nutritional deficiencies. Ask your pediatrician if you think your child needs a vitamin.

CHAPTER FIFTEEN
ADDICTION TO FOOD

ADDICTION TO SWEETS

Sugar and high-fructose corn syrup are the main characters in our love affair of all things sweet. Sugar has addictive qualities. Sugar triggers the release of dopamine, the pleasure hormone, in the brain. Some people, based on genetic differences, need more sugar to trigger the same amount of dopamine; others produce less dopamine the more sugar they eat, creating a cycle of binging to achieve the same level of dopamine in their brain, followed by withdrawal and craving.[13]

We have great campaigns, such as DARE, directed at children to prevent drug abuse. I think most parents would agree that we would not give our children any type of addictive drug. Well, then, let's include sugar in that list—no drugs and NO SUGAR. We'll create a new logo: SHARE—Sugar and High-fructose corn syrup Abuse Resistance Education.

ADDICTION TO FAT

Animal studies show similar effects with high fat junk food. In one study, rats were given access to both high fat junk food and regular food 24 hours of the day. Junk food led to compulsive eating caused by diminishing levels of dopamine release on a continuous high fat diet. The rats chose to eat junk food and get electric shocks rather than eat healthy food that was also available.[14] The proliferation of dealers of junk food—the fast food industry—makes more sense when we look at this reaction.

The really tough part is that while you can completely exclude drugs from your pantry, excluding sugar and fat is much more difficult. And so I fall back to my Mediterranean roots and say, "Pan metron ariston" or "Everything in moderation." Parents have a special responsibility when it comes to their children's diet. Since children don't shop for themselves, parents are responsible for providing healthy food and for helping children to eat appropriate portions of food. To do that, it helps to learn what that is. Lots of food and lots of junk food doesn't demonstrate parental love. While feeding and nurturing are related, overfeeding is not an act of love.

CHAPTER SIXTEEN
THE POWER OF PEER GROUPS

We all know about the power of peer groups. We think that children are affected by their peers more than they are affected by their parents. Children who spend more time with their parents are less likely to use drugs and engage in early sexual activity. What does this have to do with nutrition? What is the most common time to sit and talk with your children? The dinner table. Parents invest tremendous amounts of time taking their children to activities like sports, scouts, etc. Our children have busier calendars than we do. We have traded time for activities for time spent cooking and time spent sharing food. Eating together is one of those basic, mundane activities that enrich your family. Sit down together, turn off the television, and give your children the space to express their ideas. Eat slowly, serve small portions of food, and linger a little at the dinner table. It is time well spent.

There will be days when your children will barely offer more than a syllable in response to a question and there will be other days that they will surprise you with conversation. In our texting world, conversation is a dying art. It takes practice. The benefit is that you are less likely to gobble your food if you are taking part in an interesting conversation. That extra time lets your brain register that you are full. Devouring food quickly doesn't allow the message to descend from your brain: "STOP EATING! I am comfortably full and any more food will make me feel incredibly stuffed and ready to explode!"

Speaking of peer groups, there is a growing body of research looking at peer groups for adults. We are as affected by our peers as our children are. People who are overweight are more likely to have friends that are over-weight.[15] People who smoke are more likely to have friends who smoke. Quitting smoking is more likely if your friends, partner, or wife/husband are also trying or have quit. There is nothing particularly astounding about this observation. We are attracted to like-minded people who make us feel comfortable with ourselves. Change is a difficult proposition for adults but it is important to end the cycle of passing bad eating habits on to children.

CHAPTER SEVENTEEN
OBESITY AND
DIABETES IN CHILDREN

We know that when the body reaches an obese weight, it is very resistant to change. For adults, losing weight using diet pills usually means following a very low-calorie diet. Once the diet pills go away, it becomes much more difficult to eat small amounts of food and most people gradually regain all the weight lost. Weight loss surgery has more lasting effects and can resolve high blood pressure and diabetes. Surgery and diet pills are not an option for growing children, however. There is no substitute for them other than changing the way they eat and increasing the calories they burn by being more active. The body is actually less resistant to gradual and consistent weight loss. Doing that means changing your relationship to food permanently. For children, the stakes are higher.

Being overweight in childhood makes you much more likely to be an overweight adult. We are now seeing diabetes in children and heart disease in young adults. The health consequences of childhood obesity are overwhelming. Type-2 diabetes is the kind that is usually related to being overweight. This condition in children does not respond as well to the pills we use for type-2 diabetes in adults.[16] Diabetic children are likely to need insulin more quickly than adults, who can take diabetic pills for years before needing insulin.

Preventing diabetes in children is a national emergency that begins at your dinner table.

But how do we help overweight children to change?

A study published in Pediatrics in 2005 assessed a program of combined diet and exercise intervention in obese children and adolescents. Kids participated in supervised activity twice a week, and exercised once a week on their own. Both children and parents had nutritional education by doctors and nutritionists for 3 months. Both at the end of 3 months and at the end of a year, the children had lost weight and maintained a higher level of activity.[17] This is the model that FITKIDS brings to the table. It is the combined focus on both nutrition and exercise that is essential.

CHAPTER EIGHTEEN
EATING OUT

Did you see the movie *Supersize Me*? It generated lots of discussion. Regulating your food and caloric intake is almost impossible if you eat out on a regular basis. Fast food is, unfortunately, cheap. Restaurant food is not as cheap but is still affordable for most Americans. So eating out has become a national pastime. Consuming a whole day's worth of calories at one meal is a common practice. Food that is high in fat and sugar makes overeating more likely because of its addictive quality.

Studies prove that you are more likely to be overweight if you regularly eat fast food.[18] Furthermore, if you live in an area with a high concentration of fast food restaurants, you are more likely to be overweight.[19]

The fast food industry is making changes to bring healthier food to their menus. Restaurant chains are following suit. Calorie and nutritional information is now becoming available and we should all be using it. The calorie counts are stunning. My favorite quesadilla explosion salad at Chili's contains thirteen hundred calories—more than the total calories I consume in a typical day. The kids' portions of food are equally stunning in their caloric content. I suggest that you and your children either share or eat half portions of food when eating out. Even more, I suggest you limit eating out.

CHAPTER NINETEEN
THE IMPORTANCE OF SLEEP

I have a final topic that is really important to discuss. While this topic isn't about food, it has a lot to do with nutrition—and it is important. Children need lots of sleep. The recommendation for seven- to twelve-year-old children is ten to eleven hours and for twelve- to eighteen-year-olds, eight to nine hours nightly. During sleep, your metabolism has time to regulate itself. Inadequate sleep is tied to higher rates of obesity in children.[20]

I know that in my house, getting my boys to bed at a reasonable time is always a challenge. The more activities scheduled, the harder it is. I can definitely tell when my kids are not sleeping enough: they tend to be sluggish, irritable, and have trouble waking up—just like me. So remember to encourage kids to go to bed at a reasonable hour. A quiet, dark room is best for sleeping. Take out the television, Xbox or cell phone from the bedroom. Your children will be rested, their metabolism will function better, their performance at school will improve, and they will be happier. On that note, I wish you a restful sleep and good dreams.

CHAPTER TWENTY
THIRTY DAYS OF YUMMY EATING FOR A BUSY FAMILY

by Chrisoula Kiriazis, MD

The final part of our book is to make it as simple as possible to eat well. We are given lots of contradictory information on what kind of eating plan we should be following:

High-fat, low-fat, no-carb, low-carb. Research recently published in *JAMA* (the *Journal of the American Medical Association*) shows that, for adults, the low-glycemic diet is the healthiest approach to maintaining a healthy weight.[21] Low-glycemic diets consist of 40 percent carbohydrates in the form of whole grains, fruit, vegetables, nuts, and seeds— 40 percent fat and 20 percent protein. This guideline is in line with dietary recommendations for children and adolescents published by the American Heart Association.

How do we eat as a family if children, who are growing, can eat more? I tend to follow a low-glycemic menu—I rarely serve white rice, white potatoes, or white bread for dinner. I limit pasta to once a week and use spelt pasta some of the time. We eat lots of fruit and vegetables. Vegetables are raw, steamed, or microwaved. Fruit for breakfast is a must. We eat fat but I limit red meat to once per week. This allows my husband and me to maintain a reasonable weight. Our children eat more than we do, usually in the form of snacks and also desserts. We try to make most of those snacks healthy, though they do eat their share of sugar. Fortunately, they burn all those calories and are healthy and slim.

When I was a teenager, I went from running track and doing gymnastics to studying all the time. I continued to eat like an athlete and started gaining weight. It took me a year or two to realize that I couldn't eat as much if I exercised less. This is a message I give my boys. Their caloric intake needs to match their physical activity. The less they exercise, the less they will be able to eat. Even if they eat snacks and dessert, most of those should be healthy. So while families eat together, they don't necessarily eat the same amounts of the same things.

Here are the logistics to finding an eating plan that works for your family. You need to shop at least once a week, though it is helpful to buy fresh fruit and vegetables between your main shopping trips. Using a produce stand with locally produced fruits and vegetables is often cheaper.

Planning for dinner in the morning allows you to defrost any food you might need. I have included my favorite recipes adapted from *Cooking Light* and *Southern Living*. They have all passed the kid test with Winchester and Zachary. The weekday recipes are quick (they take between thirty and sixty minutes) and the weekend recipes take a little more time. I generally make a protein and a vegetable for dinner. Examples of snacks and desserts, including Brandon's Trail Mix Delight, are included (most adults can't eat a dessert other than fruit more than once or twice a week unless they do lots of exercise). Growing teenagers can eat a larger portion at mealtimes.

This is a real-life menu but it's just a starting point. If you are not a fan of spices, use less. Alter the recipes, take out the avocados, change the sides—make it yours. Keep experimenting with new foods and new recipes. There are splurge days included, usually on the weekend. On those days, you can eat anything you want, usually in moderate quantities, and that should make you happy :). BON APPETIT!

BREAKFAST ON WEEKDAYS

½-cup of whole-grain cereal, like Raisin Bran, Mueslix, or Great Grains with low- or non-fat milk or low-fat vanilla soymilk
   or
½-cup regular old-fashioned oats with raisins, dried cranberries, or cherries and a sprinkling of nuts (cooked for 3 minutes in the microwave). Add low-fat milk or low-fat vanilla soymilk, brown sugar, or maple syrup to your taste.
   or
1 cup of yogurt (Fage or Chobani are our favorites) with a sprinkling of nuts and granola or whole-grain cereal
   Sprinkle all of the above with cinnamon, which helps regulate blood sugar and may improve memory function.

Add ½-cup of fruit of any kind and/or ½-glass of orange juice.

BREAKFAST ON WEEKENDS

If you are not hurried, it's a great time to make omelets (experiment with the add-ons), scrambled eggs, French toast (1 or 2 slices), pancakes, or Belgian waffles. My kids love boxed Eggo Cinnamon toast waffles (no more than 2) when we are hurried.
   Add a slice of bacon if you like.
   Always include a fruit of your choice.
   Kids should drink milk—either low-fat or soymilk.

LUNCH ON WEEKDAYS and WEEKENDS

Leftovers are always a good choice. Add fruit for dessert.

A sandwich using whole-grain sandwich thins with one slice of cheese and 2 or 3 slices of lean meat with some lettuce and either mayo or mustard, or both
Raw carrots, slices of cucumber for a side dish
A fruit like an apple for dessert
    or
Cheese quesadilla made with low-carb tortillas stuffed with any cheese you like—usually 1 slice of cheese and a sprinkling of low-fat mozzarella. (Takes 3 minutes to cook on a quesadilla maker.)
Serve with salsa and side of fruit.
    or
Peanut or almond butter and jam on whole-grain bread Serve with any fruit you like.

SNACKS

A small bowl of whole-grain tortilla chips with salsa
    or
Fruit
    or
Unsalted almonds with Nutella
    or
Trail mix
    or
Sunrise energy bars or energy bar of your choice
    or
Carrots with hummus

DESSERTS

½-cup ice cream or frozen yogurt
    or

1–2 cookies
   or
anything you like in small amounts

PIZZA NIGHT

Our current favorites are Palermo's Thin Crust Margherita and Chicken Fajita Pizza. We usually eat one pizza among the four of us. Add any other veggies you like.

You can buy pizza. Thin-crust pizza without pepperoni or sausage is healthier.

You can make pizza with Mama Mary's Pizza Crusts that are precooked. Add your own sauce and toppings and cook for 10 minutes.

DINNER MENUS—Recipes are attached.

Day 1 Monday chicken cobb salad
Day 2 Tuesday tuna melts
Day 3 Wednesday pork loin chops with green beans
Day 4 Thursday mac and cheese, served with raw carrots
Day 5 Friday dinner—pizza night
Day 6 Saturday dinner—splurge night/dinner out
Day 7 Sunday dinner—steak with sweet potato fries, romaine salad

Day 8 Monday tilapia piccata served with snow peas
Day 9 Tuesday subway night—six-inch subway sandwiches with whole-wheat bread and lots of veggies
Day 10 Wednesday sesame crusted salmon with cucumbers
Day 11 Thursday Mediterranean turkey burgers with a salad
Day 12 Friday pizza night
Day 13 Saturday linguine with meat sauce or meatballs, served with salad
Day 14 Sunday dinner out

Day 15 Monday spice-crusted salmon with cucumber relish
Day 16 Tuesday tuna melts
Day 17 Wednesday chicken piccata with spinach fettuccine
Day 18 Thursday flank steak with quinoa and brown rice
Day 19 Friday dinner out
Day 20 Saturday fish tacos with broccoli slaw
Day 21 Sunday pork tenderloin with fig glaze, asparagus on the side

Day 22 Monday leftover pork with brown or wild rice
Day 23 Tuesday crisp-crusted catfish with green beans
Day 24 Wednesday turkey taco salad
Day 25 Thursday dinner out
Day 26 Friday pizza night
Day 27 Saturday chicken Parmesan with a side salad
Day 28 Sunday lamb chops with mashed sweet potatoes and asparagus

Day 29 Monday quinoa with chicken, orange, and avocado
Day 30 Tuesday baked fish with chipotle butter, steamed broccoli

RECIPE INDEX

Linguine with Meat Sauce

⅄ 2 pounds lean ground beef
⅄ 1 medium onion
⅄ 2 garlic cloves, minced
⅄ 1 (28-ounce) can crushed tomatoes
⅄ 1 (8-ounce) can tomato sauce
⅄ 1 (6-ounce) can tomato paste
⅄ 1 teaspoon salt
⅄ 2 teaspoons sugar
⅄ 1 stick cinnamon
⅄ 8 ounces cooked linguine

Preparation

1. Sauté onion and garlic in a Dutch oven for 4-5 minutes, until onion is soft.
2. Stir in beef and cook, stirring continuously until it is no longer pink.
3. Stir in tomatoes and next 4 ingredients. Add cinnamon stick.
4. Simmer 30 minutes. Set mixture aside.
5. Cook pasta while beef is simmering.
6. Serve with a side salad of romaine lettuce with cucumbers, tomato, olives, carrots, seasoned with apple cider vinegar, olive oil, and salt drizzled on top. Experiment with the amounts you like.

Baked Macaroni and Cheese

Ingredients

- 2 cups cooked elbow pasta
- 3 tablespoons butter
- 3 tablespoons all-purpose flour
- 2 cups fat-free milk
- 1 small onion
- 4 slices of bacon, cooked in the microwave and patted dry with paper towels
- 2 cups sharp cheddar cheese
- 3 ounces low-fat cream cheese with chives and onions, softened
- ½-teaspoon salt and 1/8-teaspoon pepper
- 1/8-cup panko bread crumbs

Preparation

1. Preheat oven to 350°. Prepare elbow pasta according to package directions.
2. Sauté onion in a Dutch oven for 5 minutes.
3. Cook bacon in the microwave and chop when done.
4. Meanwhile, melt 3 tbsp butter in a Dutch oven over medium heat.
5. Gradually whisk in flour; cook, whisking constantly, for 1 minute.
6. Gradually whisk in milk until smooth; cook, whisking constantly, for 8 to 10 minutes or until slightly thickened.
7. Whisk in cheddar cheese, cream cheese, salt, and red pepper until smooth.
8. Remove from heat, and stir in bacon and onion.

9. Pour pasta into an 8-x-8-inch Pyrex dish coated with cooking spray. Sprinkle with panko bread crumbs and smoked paprika.
10. Bake at 350° for 20 minutes or until golden and bubbly. Let stand 5 minutes before serving.
11. Serve with raw baby carrots.

Baked Fish with Chipotle Butter

Ingredients
- ½-teaspoon ground cumin
- ½-teaspoon smoked paprika
- ¼-teaspoon salt
- 1/8-teaspoon black pepper
- 4 (6-ounce) red snapper, flounder, tilapia, or fillets
- Cooking spray
- 1 tablespoon butter, softened
- 1 canned chipotle chili in adobo sauce, finely minced
- 1 tablespoon fresh lime juice
- Lime wedges

Preparation
Preheat oven to 400°.

Combine cumin, paprika, salt, and pepper; sprinkle over fish. Place fish on a baking sheet coated with cooking spray; bake 15 minutes or until fish flakes easily.

While fish bakes, combine butter, lime juice, and chili. Spread mixture evenly over fish.

Serve with steamed broccoli.

Spicy Chicken Breasts with Tomato-Avocado Salad

Ingredients

- 4 (6-ounce) skinless, boneless chicken breast halves
- 1 tablespoon paprika
- 1 teaspoon ground cumin
- 1 teaspoon dried oregano
- ¾-teaspoon sugar
- ¾-teaspoon garlic powder
- ½-teaspoon salt
- ½-teaspoon dried thyme
- ¼-teaspoon ground red pepper
- 1 tablespoon fresh lime juice
- 1 ripe peeled avocado, cut into 16 slices
- 2 tomatoes, cut into small pieces
- ¼-cup finely chopped red onion
- ¼-cup corn
- ½-cup black beans
- Rice wine vinegar, olive oil, and salt to taste

Preparation

Combine paprika and next 7 ingredients (through pepper) in a small bowl. Sprinkle paprika mixture evenly over chicken; cook chicken in a Cuisinart grill—7 minutes for each 2 chicken breasts or in a pan, cooking 4 minutes on each side or until done. Let chicken stand for 5 minutes before cutting crosswise into ¼-inch-thick slices.

Combine juice and remaining ingredients in a bowl, tossing to coat with dressing. Heat a grill pan over medium-high heat. Coat pan with cooking spray. Grill avocado 2 minutes on each side or until well-marked; remove from pan.

Serve 1 chicken breast with tomato avocado salad.

Greek Chicken Cobb Salad

Ingredients

- Olive oil to coat pan
- 4 chicken breasts
- Grill Creations St. Louis Style Smokey Mesquite seasoning to taste
- 1 diced peeled avocado
- 2 tablespoons sliced red onions
- 1 carrot, peeled and sliced
- 1/3-cup Café Athens Greek feta dressing
- 2 tablespoons crumbled feta cheese
- 2 bacon slices, cooked and crumbled
- Romaine lettuce
- Caesar croutons

Preparation

Heat a large nonstick skillet over medium-high heat. Coat pan with olive oil. Sprinkle chicken with mesquite dressing. Add chicken to pan; cook 5 minutes on each side or until done. Cut into ½-inch slices.

Combine romaine lettuce, tomatoes, carrots, avocado, and onions in a large bowl. Add chicken slices, bacon, and croutons. Drizzle mixture with dressing; toss gently to coat.

Chicken Parmesan

Ingredients

- 1 cup Italian-seasoned breadcrumbs
- 2 tablespoons all-purpose flour
- ½-teaspoon ground red pepper
- 6–8 chicken tenders or 4 chicken breasts divided in half
- 2 egg whites, lightly beaten
- 1 small package portabella mushrooms, sliced
- 1 package sautéed spinach
- Handful of chopped olives
- Salt, pepper, and garlic powder
- 1 tablespoon olive oil
- Bottled tomato sauce of your choice
- 1 cup shredded mozzarella cheese
- ¼-cup freshly grated parmesan cheese

Preparation

Sauté mushrooms in olive oil.

Sauté spinach in same pan and sprinkle with salt, pepper, and garlic powder to taste.

Combine breadcrumbs, flour, and ground red pepper in a small bowl.

Dip 1 chicken breast in egg whites, and coat with breadcrumb mixture.
Dip again in egg mixture, and coat again in breadcrumb mixture.

Repeat procedure with the remaining chicken.

Cook chicken in hot oil over medium heat 2 to 3 minutes on each side or until done.

Place chicken breasts in a single layer in a lightly greased 8-inch square baking dish. Top evenly with mushrooms, spinach, olives, tomato sauce, and cheeses. Bake at 350° for 20 minutes or until cheese melts.

You can omit the mushroom, spinach, and olives if your children object.

Serve with salad of your choice.

Chicken Piccata with Capers

Ingredients

- 4 (6-ounce) skinless, boneless chicken breast halves
- ¼-cup all-purpose flour (about 1 ounce)
- 1 tablespoon olive oil
- 1 cup chicken broth
- 2 tablespoons fresh lemon juice
- 2 tablespoons capers
- 1 clove minced fresh garlic
- 1 package of small, sautéed portabella mushrooms
- ¼-teaspoon salt
- ¼-teaspoon freshly ground black pepper
- 4 cups hot cooked spinach fettuccine, whole-wheat, or spelt pasta

Preparation

Cut chicken into small pieces and mix in a Ziploc bag with salt, pepper, and flour.

Heat butter and oil in a large skillet over medium-high heat. Add chicken, and cook for 3 minutes on each side or until browned.

Add chicken broth, mushrooms, lemon juice, capers, and garlic to pan; simmer for 15–20 minutes.

Cook pasta according to package instructions.

Serve chicken over pasta. Top with sauce from pan and parmesan cheese.

Make a salad or serve with raw carrots.

Crisp-Crusted Catfish

Ingredients

- 2 tablespoons light ranch dressing or dressing of your choice
- 2 large egg whites
- 6 tablespoons yellow cornmeal
- ¼-cup (1 ounce) grated fresh parmesan cheese
- 2 tablespoons all-purpose flour
- ¼-teaspoon ground red pepper
- 1/8-teaspoon salt
- 4 (6-ounce) farm-raised catfish fillets
- Olive oil and cooking spray
- 4 lemon wedges
- Green beans

Preparation

Preheat oven to 425°.

Combine the dressing and egg whites in a small bowl, stirring well with a whisk. Combine the cornmeal, cheese, flour, pepper, and salt in a shallow dish. Dip fish in egg white mixture and then in the cornmeal mixture.

Place fish on a baking sheet coated with cooking spray; bake at 425° for 12 minutes on each side or until lightly browned and fish flakes easily when tested with a fork. Drizzle with fresh lemon from wedges.

Steam green beans for 17 minutes or until crisp in a steamer.

Serve fish with steamed green beans drizzled with olive oil and a sprinkle of salt.

Cumin-Spiced Fish
Tacos with Avocado-Mango Salsa

Ingredients

- 1 tablespoon cumin seeds
- ¾-teaspoon salt, divided
- ½-teaspoon paprika
- ¼-teaspoon freshly ground black pepper
- 2 garlic cloves, minced
- 6–8 pieces of tilapia fillets
- 1 tablespoon canola oil
- 1 cup sliced peeled avocado

- 2/3-cup finely chopped peeled ripe mango
- ¼-cup chopped green onions
- ¼-cup finely chopped red onion
- 2 tablespoons finely chopped fresh cilantro
- 1 tablespoon fresh lime juice
- ¼-teaspoon ground red pepper
- 8 (6-inch) wheat tortillas
- Low-fat sour cream, optional

Preparation

1. Toast cumin seeds in your toaster for 2 minutes or so. Place cumin, ½-teaspoon salt, paprika, and black pepper in a spice grinder or use a mortar and pestle to process until finely ground. If you are rushed, used ground cumin.
   Combine cumin mixture and garlic; rub over fish.
   Return the skillet to medium-high heat. Add oil to pan; swirl to coat.
   Add fish; cook 2 minutes on each side or until done. Remove from heat; keep warm.

2. Combine the remaining ¼-teaspoon salt, avocado, and next 6 ingredients (through ¼-teaspoon red pepper).

3. Heat tortillas according to package instructions. Break fish into pieces; divide evenly among tortillas. Top each tortilla with 2 tablespoons salsa. Add sour cream if you like. Fold tortillas in half; serve immediately.

On a weeknight when I make fish tacos, I use ground cumin instead of cumin seeds. Instead of making the salsa in the recipe, I put out sides of bottled salsa, sour cream, and guacamole.

Serve with store-bought broccoli slaw sprinkled with salt and drizzled with rice wine vinegar and olive oil. Add a little mayo or salad dressing of your choice if you prefer.

Flank Steak with Mango Chutney

Ingredients

⋏ Steak:
⋏ 1 tablespoon brown sugar
⋏ 1 teaspoon salt
⋏ ¾-teaspoon ground cumin
⋏ 3 garlic cloves, minced
⋏ 1 (1½-pound) flank steak, trimmed
⋏ Cooking spray

⋏ Chutney:
⋏ 1 peeled ripe mango, diced
⋏ 1 teaspoon olive oil
⋏ 1 cup thinly vertically sliced onion
⋏ 1 tablespoon minced peeled fresh ginger
⋏ 1/3-cup cider vinegar
⋏ 2 tablespoons brown sugar
⋏ 2 tablespoons fresh lime juice
⋏ ¼-teaspoon salt
⋏ 1½ tablespoons chopped fresh cilantro
⋏ Lime wedges (optional)
⋏ Seeds of Change quinoa and brown rice in a microwave packet.

Preparation

Prepare grill or preheat broiler.

To prepare steak, combine first 4 ingredients. Sprinkle steak evenly with sugar mixture. Place steak on grill rack coated with cooking spray; grill or broil for 6 minutes on each side or until desired degree of doneness.

Let stand 10 minutes. Cut steak diagonally across grain into thin slices.

Heat oil in a small saucepan over medium-high heat. Add onion; sauté 4 minutes. Add ginger; sauté 1 minute. Add vinegar, 2 tablespoons sugar, juice, ¼-teaspoon salt, and pepper; cook 5 minutes or until liquid almost evaporates. Stir in chopped mango; cook 1 minute. Remove from heat. Stir in cilantro. Add lime wedges, if desired.

On a weeknight, I often make this steak without the chutney in the broiler. You can add a little barbecue sauce of your choice if you like.

Microwave quinoa and brown rice for 90 seconds. Serve with steak.

Tilapia Piccata with Spinach or Snow Peas

Ingredients
- ¼-teaspoon salt, divided
- 1/8-teaspoon black pepper, divided
- 4 tilapia fillets
- 2 tablespoons all-purpose flour
- 2 teaspoons olive oil

- 1/3-cup dry white wine
- 2 tablespoons fresh lemon juice
- 1 tablespoon drained capers, chopped
- 2 tablespoons butter
- 4 cups fresh baby spinach
- Snow peas

Preparation
1. Sprinkle fish with ¼-teaspoon salt and remaining 1/8-teaspoon pepper. Dredge fish in flour.
2. Heat oil in a large nonstick skillet over medium-high heat. Add fish to pan; cook 3–5 minutes on each side or until fish flakes easily when tested with a fork.
3. Add wine, juice, and capers to pan; cook 1 minute. Add butter to pan, stirring until butter melts. Pour sauce over fish.
4. Add spinach to pan; sauté 1 minute or until wilted.
5. Serve fish with spinach.

My children don't like sautéed spinach yet, so for them I serve the fish with snow peas. To prepare snow peas, cut the top edge and peel the hard part of the spine off. Microwave for 3 minutes, stopping and stirring after 1½ minutes. Drizzle with olive oil and lightly sprinkle with salt.

Mediterranean Turkey Burgers

Ingredients
- ½-cup panko bread crumbs
- ¼-cup (1 ounce) crumbled feta cheese
- 1 tablespoon minced red onion
- 1 lightly beaten egg
- 2 tablespoons store-bought pesto (I like the pesto with pine nuts and almonds.)
- ¼-teaspoon freshly ground black pepper

- 1 pound ground turkey breast
- 1 garlic clove, minced
- Cooking spray
- 4 cups romaine, 1 tomato, ½ cucumber, sliced baby carrots, olives, and crumbled feta
- For dressing: salt, olive oil, and balsamic vinegar in desired amounts

Preparation
1. Combine first 8 ingredients in a bowl; mix until combined. Divide panko mixture into 4 portions, shaping each into a ½-inch-thick oval patty.
2. Heat your broiler. Coat pan with cooking spray. Broil for 7 minutes on each side or until done.
3. Serve turkey burgers with a salad.
4. If you have time and would like, make tzatziki sauce: combine ½-cup plain low-fat Greek-style yogurt; ¼-cup finely chopped seeded cucumber; ¼-teaspoon salt; and 1/8-teaspoon ground red pepper.

Meatballs with Linguine

Ingredients
- 1 cup finely chopped onion
- ¼-cup dry breadcrumbs
- ½-teaspoon kosher salt
- ½-teaspoon dill seeds
- 1/8-teaspoon freshly ground black pepper
- 1 pound ground round or sirloin
- 1 large egg white, lightly beaten
- Cooking spray
- Bottled marinara

Preparation
To prepare meatballs, combine first 7 ingredients in a bowl; shape mixture into meatballs. Bake at 400° for 20 minutes in a pan coated with cooking spray.

Prepare linguine according to instructions.

Top with meatballs and your favorite bottled marinara, which has been heated in the microwave or on stove top.

Pepper, Coriander, and Sesame Seed-Crusted Salmon

Ingredients

- 1 tablespoon sesame seeds
- 1 teaspoon black peppercorns
- 1 teaspoon coriander seeds
- ¼-teaspoon salt
- 4 (6-ounce) salmon fillets, skinned (about 1-inch thick)

- 1 teaspoon olive oil
- 2/3-cup apricot nectar
- ½-cup diced red bell pepper
- ¼-cup cider vinegar
- 1 teaspoon minced peeled fresh ginger

Preparation

Combine first 4 ingredients and crush with a mortar and pestle. If you are rushed, used ground coriander and pepper and leave the sesame seeds unground. Place seed mixture in a large shallow dish. Coat 1 side of each fillet with seed mixture.

Heat oil in a large nonstick skillet over medium-high heat. Add fillets, seed sides down; sauté 4 minutes on each side or until fish flakes easily when tested with a fork. Remove fish from pan.

Add apricot nectar and the remaining ingredients to pan, and bring to a boil, scraping pan to loosen browned bits. Cook 1 minute. Reduce heat; return fish to pan. Baste with nectar mixture. Cover and simmer 1 minute.

You can also broil the salmon for 10–15 minutes depending on the thickness, and make the sauce while the salmon is cooking. The results are very similar and it is faster.

Serve with cucumber slices, sprinkled with salt.

Pork Loin Chops with Red Currant Sauce

Ingredients

- ½-teaspoon dried thyme
- ½-teaspoon salt
- ¼-teaspoon smoked paprika
- ¼-teaspoon dried rubbed sage
- 1/8-teaspoon black pepper

- 6–8 pork loin chops, no more than ½-inch thick
- Olive oil
- 1/3-cup red currant jelly
- 3 tablespoons cider vinegar
- 2 tablespoons chopped fresh chives

Preparation

1. Combine first 5 ingredients in a small bowl. Rub pork chops with spice mixture.
2. Heat a large nonstick skillet over medium-high heat. Coat pan with olive oil. Add pork to pan, and cook for 3 minutes on each side. Remove pork from pan; keep warm.
3. Heat red currant jelly and cider vinegar on the stove top or in the microwave. Add chives. I often omit the sauce when making this recipe on weeknights. The pork chops are delicious without it.
4. Serve with steamed green beans sprinkled with sliced almonds, and drizzled with olive oil. Sprinkle with salt if you like.

Quinoa Salad with Chicken, Avocado, and Oranges

Ingredients

- 1¼ cups quinoa
- 1 teaspoon chili powder
- 3 teaspoons minced garlic, divided
- Zest of 1 lime
- 2 teaspoons plus 3 tbsp olive oil
- 1 teaspoon kosher salt, divided

- 1 teaspoon pepper, divided
- 1 pound boned, skinned chicken thighs
- ¼-cup lime juice
- ½-cup chopped fresh cilantro
- 4 large oranges, peeled and segmented
- 2 ripe avocados, peeled and cubed

Preparation

1. Cook quinoa according to package directions and fluff with a fork.
   Transfer to a large bowl and cool. Use the refrigerator or freezer to cool the quinoa to speed things up.
2. Preheat broiler. In a large bowl, stir together chili powder, 2 tsp garlic, lime zest, 2 tsp oil, and ½-tsp each salt and pepper. Add chicken and toss to coat.
   Put chicken on a baking sheet and broil, turning once, until browned and cooked through, about 12 minutes total.
   The alternative is to use a kitchen grill—like the Foreman or Cuisinart grill—to cook the chicken. You can skip the dressing entirely and use a spice rub of

your liking. My favorite, also used in the cobb salad, is Durkee's St. Louis Style Smokey Mesquite Seasoning. Let the chicken cool slightly.

3. Add remaining ingredients to quinoa and chicken; toss to coat.

   You can trade oranges for cherry tomatoes and add feta cheese instead of avocados; use parsley in place of cilantro for a Mediterranean twist.

Simply Great Steak with Sweet Potato Fries
(The spices in this steak recipe come from Bobby Flay.)

Ingredients
- 2 ribeye steaks (about 1½ inches thick), cut in half
- Salt and pepper
- Cayenne
- Chipotle chili powder
- Olive oil

- Fries:
- 1 teaspoon sea or kosher salt
- 2 teaspoons paprika
- 1 teaspoon coarsely ground black pepper
- ½-teaspoon garlic powder
- ½-teaspoon onion powder
- ½-teaspoon chili powder
- 1 teaspoon olive oil
- 4 medium sweet potatoes, each cut into 12 wedges or slices

Preparation
To prepare steak, coat steak with spices (in the amounts you like) and drizzle with olive oil. Cover and wrap steak in Saran Wrap, place in refrigerator for at least 30 minutes but even as long as many hours, if you like. You will be surprised that the spice is mild when this steak is cooked.

Prepare grill with one side on medium heat and one side on high heat.

Remove steak from refrigerator and let stand at room temperature for 15 minutes. Place steak on grill rack coated with cooking spray over high heat; grill 3 minutes on each side. Turn steak and place over medium heat; grill 3 minutes on each side or until desired degree of doneness.

To prepare fries, chop the potatoes and place them on a pan coated with cooking spray. Sprinkle the spices on top. I rarely measure them anymore but just use as much as I like. Toss gently to coat.

Place potatoes on grill rack coated with cooking spray over medium heat; grill 18 minutes or until sweet potatoes are tender, turning occasionally.

You can also bake these on a foil-lined sheet at 425° for about 20 minutes or so. Turn them halfway through.

Make a salad to accompany this meal.

Spice-Rubbed Pork
Tenderloin with Fig-Chili Glaze

Ingredients
⊿ Pork:
⊿ 1 teaspoon brown sugar
⊿ ¾-teaspoon chili powder
⊿ ¾-teaspoon paprika
⊿ ½-teaspoon salt
⊿ ½-teaspoon onion powder
⊿ ½-teaspoon ground cumin
⊿ ¼-teaspoon garlic powder
⊿ ¼-teaspoon dried thyme

⊿ 1 (1-pound) pork tenderloin, trimmed
⊿ Olive oil

⊿ Fig-Chili Glaze:
⊿ ½-cup fig preserves
⊿ ¼-cup rice wine vinegar
⊿ 1 tablespoon low-sodium soy sauce
⊿ ¼-teaspoon salt
⊿ 1 tablespoon chili paste with garlic (omit this if you don't like spice)

Preparation
Preheat oven to 425°.

To prepare pork, combine first 8 ingredients in a small bowl. Rub pork tenderloin with spice mixture and drizzle with olive oil; refrigerate for 20 minutes.

Place pork on a pan coated with cooking spray. Bake at 425° for 20 minutes or until meat thermometer registers 160°. Let stand 5 minutes; cut into ¼-inch-thick slices.

While the pork is cooking, microwave or steam asparagus until crisp or tender.

To prepare glaze, combine the ingredients and microwave for 2–3 minutes.
Serve glaze with pork and asparagus.

Spice-Rubbed Salmon with Cucumber Relish

Ingredients
- 1 tablespoon brown sugar
- 1 teaspoon garlic powder
- 1 teaspoon dried oregano
- 1 teaspoon ground cumin
- 1 teaspoon chili powder
- 1 teaspoon paprika
- ½-teaspoon salt, divided
- ¼-teaspoon dried thyme

- 4 (6-ounce) salmon fillets, skinned
- Cooking spray
- 2 cups chopped cucumber
- ½-cup chopped red bell pepper
- ¼-cup onion
- 2 tablespoons chopped fresh cilantro
- 1 tablespoon capers
- 1 tablespoon cider vinegar

Preparation

Preheat broiler.

Combine first 6 ingredients, ¼-teaspoon salt, and dried thyme; rub evenly over fish. Place fish on a pan coated with cooking spray. Broil 8–12 minutes or until fish flakes easily when tested with a fork.

Combine ¼-teaspoon salt, cucumber, and remaining ingredients; serve with fish.

If you are rushed, drizzle fish with a little maple syrup and serve with cucumber slices or sliced cherry tomatoes.

Tuna Melts

Ingredients

- 2½ tablespoons olive oil
- 2 tablespoons thinly sliced shallots (onions or scallions are fine too)
- 1 tablespoon Dijon mustard
- ¼-teaspoon black pepper
- 1/8-teaspoon salt
- 3 (6-ounce) cans chunk light tuna in water, drained and flaked
- 1½ tablespoons fresh lemon juice
- 1 avocado
- 1 cup cherry tomatoes, quartered
- 1 cup broccoli slaw
- Spinach leaves
- 1/3-cup shredded muenster cheese or cheese of your choice
- Slices of pumpernickel or whole-grain bread

Preparation

1. Combine first 6 ingredients in a medium bowl, stirring well to coat. Peel and chop avocado. Add avocado, broccoli slaw, lemon juice, and tomatoes to tuna mixture; toss well to combine.
2. Place spinach leaves on bread, cover with cheese slices, and toast in a toaster oven until cheese melts.
3. Place 1 bread slice, cheese side up, on each of 4 plates, and divide tuna mixture evenly among bread slices.

You can exchange avocado for olives or edamame beans and use mayo instead of olive oil if you prefer.

Turkey and Spaghetti Squash Enchiladas

Ingredients
- 2 spaghetti squash
- 2 tablespoons olive oil
- 1 small chopped onion
- 1 garlic clove
- ½-teaspoon salt
- 2 teaspoons ground cumin
- 2 teaspoons chili powder
- ¼-teaspoon black pepper
- 2 tablespoons tomato paste
- 1-lb ground turkey
- 8 whole-wheat or low-carb tortillas
- 1 14-oz can enchilada sauce, mild or medium to your liking
- 1–2 cups low-fat mozzarella sauce

For the spaghetti squash on the side:
- ½-teaspoon salt
- 1 cup cilantro
- 1 tablespoon olive oil
- ½-cup vegetable broth (chicken broth is fine)
- 1 tablespoon peppercorns
- 1 12-oz packet of frozen unshelled edamame
- 1 garlic clove
- 1 tbsp lime juice
- 1/8-cup feta cheese

Preparation
Preheat oven to 400°. Split spaghetti squash in half length-wise. Scoop seeds out. Line a baking sheet with foil and

coat with cooking spray. Place squash flesh down on foil and bake for 30–40 minutes. Scoop out squash when done.

Heat oil in a large nonstick skillet over medium-high heat. Add onion and garlic and sauté 5 minutes until onion is tender. Add cumin and chili powder and cook for one minute. Add turkey and cook until the meat is no longer pink, about 5 minutes. Add tomato paste, salt, and pepper. Cook for 5 minutes and then let cool.

Combine flesh from ½ of one spaghetti squash with the turkey. Wrap the mixture in tortillas and place in a baking dish coated with cooking spray. Cover with enchilada sauce and mozzarella cheese. Bake at 350° for 20 minutes.

Meanwhile, cook edamame in the microwave and shell. (Kids are great at shelling.) Combine cilantro, lime, broth, feta, salt, garlic, and edamame in a food processor.

Pulse until coarsely chopped. Serve pesto over remaining portion of spaghetti squash as a side.

Ground Turkey Taco Salad

Ingredients

- 2 tablespoons olive oil
- 1 small chopped onion
- 1 garlic clove
- ½-teaspoon salt
- 2 teaspoons ground cumin
- 2 teaspoons chili powder
- ¼-teaspoon black pepper
- 2 tablespoons tomato paste
- 1-lb ground turkey

- Romaine lettuce, 4 cups chopped carrots, diced tomatoes
- Rice wine or red wine vinegar, olive oil and salt
- Bottled salsa, shredded cheese, sour cream, and guacamole if you like

Preparation

Heat oil in a large nonstick skillet over medium-high heat. Add onion and garlic and sauté 5 minutes until onion is tender. Add cumin and chili powder and cook for 1 minute. Add turkey and cook until the meat is no longer pink, about 5 minutes. Add tomato paste, salt, and pepper. Cook for 5 minutes and then let cool.

Chop the romaine lettuce, carrots, and tomatoes. Toss with dressing. Divide in four dishes and top with turkey, salsa, cheese, sour cream, and guacamole.

This recipe works equally well with ground beef and is the same as the turkey prepared for the enchiladas.

Lamb Chops with Pomegranate Reduction

Ingredients

- Cooking spray and olive oil
- 8 (3-ounce) lamb rib chops, trimmed
- ½-teaspoon black pepper
- ¼-teaspoon salt
- ½-teaspoon chopped fresh thyme
- ½-teaspoon oregano
- ½-teaspoon garlic powder
- ¾-cup pomegranate juice
- 1 teaspoon Dijon mustard
- ½-teaspoon honey
- 2 tablespoons minced shallots
- 1 teaspoon minced garlic
- 1 teaspoon cornstarch
- 1 teaspoon water
- 1 tablespoon chopped fresh chives
- 1/8-teaspoon salt
- 1/8-teaspoon black pepper
- 3–4 sweet potatoes
- 3 tablespoons 2% milk
- Salt and pepper to taste

Preparation

1. Preheat oven to 400°.
2. Sprinkle lamb with herbs, salt, and pepper, and drizzle with olive oil.
3. Sear lamb chops in pan on high heat for no more than 2–3 minutes.
4. Coat a foil-lined baking sheet with cooking spray. Place lamb on prepared pan. Bake lamb at 400° for

20 minutes or until desired degree of doneness. Let stand for 10 minutes covered with foil before slicing.

5. Combine juice, mustard, and honey in a small bowl. Heat a small saucepan over medium-high heat. Coat pan with cooking spray. Add shallots and garlic to pan; sauté 1 minute. Stir in juice mixture; bring to a boil. Reduce heat and cook until reduced to ½ cup (about 5 minutes). Combine cornstarch and water in a small bowl; stir until smooth. Add cornstarch mixture to pan; bring to a boil. Cook 1 minute, stirring constantly. Remove from heat; stir in chives, 1/8-teaspoon salt, and 1/8-teaspoon pepper. Serve with lamb.

6. While lamb is cooking, steam sweet potatoes, mash, add milk, and season with salt and pepper.

7. Steam or microwave asparagus and serve with lamb and sweet potatoes.

8. It's not necessary to make the sauce for the lamb chops. They are delicious on their own.

Brandon's Chocolate Trail Mix Delight

Ingredients
- 1 cup dried fruit (I like banana chips and cranberries.)
- 1 cup nuts (I like dry roasted peanuts, spicy almonds, or macadamia nuts.)
- 1 cup raisins
- 1 cup dark chocolate chips (also a great substitute is peanut butter chips)

Preparation
- Mix it all together.
- Enjoy!!!

For more information on Brandon's program, go to www. BEAFITKID.org or friend us on Facebook.

A portion of the proceeds of this book will go back into the program and will help to create a scholarship fund for those kids who need this program most and can afford it least.

Let's be the change that America needs...

Footnotes:

[1] Bostrom, P. "PGC1-alpha Dependent Myokine That Drives Brown-fat like Devleopment of White Fat and Thermogenesis." *Nature.com*. Nature Publishing Group, n.d. Web. 19 Aug. 2012. <http://www.nature.com/nature/journal/vaop/ncurrent/abs/nature10777.html>.

[2] Gilsanz, Vicente. "Changes in Brown Adipose Tissue in Boys and Girls during Childhood and Puberty." *National Center for Biotechnology Information*. U.S. National Library of Medicine, n.d. Web. 19 Aug. 2012. <http://www.ncbi.nlm.nih.gov/pubmed/22048045>.

[3] Benson, A. "Muscular Strength and Cardiorespiratoy Fitness Is Associated with Higher Insulin Sensitivity in Children and Adolescents." *National Center for Biotechnology Information*. U.S. National Library of Medicine, n.d. Web. 19 Aug. 2012. <http://www.ncbi.nlm.nih.gov/pubmed/17907329>.

[4] Chaddock, L., and K.I. Erickson. "A Neuroimaging Investigation of the Association between Aerobic Fitness, Hippocampal Volume, and Memory Performance in Preadolescent Children." N.p., 22 Aug. 2010. Web.

[5] Tomporowski, Phillip D., Catherine L. Davis, and Mathew Gregoski. "Effects of Aerobic Exercise on Overweight Children's Cognitive Functioning." *Medicine & Science in Sports & Exercise* 38.Supplement (2006): S28. Web.

[6] J. N. Farr & R. M. Blew & V. R. Lee & T. G. Lohman & S. B. "Associations of Physical Activity Duration, Frequency, and Load with Volumetric BMD, Geometry, and Bone

Strength in Girls." *Osteoporos Int DOI 10.1007/s00198-010-1361-8.* (2010): n. pag. Print.

[7]Williamson, Dinkie, Alison Dewey, and Hannah Steinberg. "Mood Change through Physical Exercise in Nine to Ten-Year-old Children." *Perceptual and Motor Skills, 2001* 93 (2001): 311-16. Web.Arch Dis Child. 2009 Sep;94(9):686-9. Epub 2009 Jul 24.

[8]Nixon GM, Thompson JM, Han DY, Becroft DM, Clark PM, Robinson E, Waldie KE, Wild CJ, Black PN, Mitchell EA. Falling asleep: the determinants of sleep latency. Ritchie Centre for Baby Health Research, Monash Institute of Medical Research, Monash University, Melbourne, Australia. Sep 94(9)686-9

[9]Blimkie, CJ. "Resistance Training during Pre-and Early Puberty:efficacy, Trainiability, Mechanisms, and Persistence." *Can J Sports Sci* 4 (1992): 264-79. Web.

[10]American Academy of Pediatrics. "Strength Training by Children and Adolescents." *Pediatrics* 121: 835-40, 2008

[11]Yu, Hongjian, and Harold Goldstein. "Bubbling Over: Soda Consumption and Its Link to Obesity in California." *UCLA for Health Policy Research* (n.d.): n. pag. Sept. 2009. Web.

[12]Malik, Vasanti S., Matthias B. Schulze, and Frank B. Hu. "Intake of Sugar-sweetended Beverages and Weight Gain: A Systematic Review." *AM J Clin Nutr* 84.2 (2006 Aug): 272-88. Web.

[13]Avena, Nicole M., Pedro Rada, and Bartley G. Hoebel. "Evidence for Sugar Addiction: Behavioral and Neurochemical Effects of Intermittent, Excessive Sugar Intake." *Neuroscience & Biobehavioral Reviews* 32.1 (2008): 20-39. Web.

[14]Johnson, Paul M., and Paul J. Kenny. "Corrigendum: Dopamine D2 Receptors in Addiction-like Reward Dysfunction and Compulsive Eating in Obese Rats." *Nature Neuroscience* 13.8 (2010): 1033. Web.

[15] Christakis, Nicholas A. MD, PhD, MPH, and James H. Fowler, PhD, "The Spread of Obesity in a Large Social Network over 32 Years." N Engl J Med, 357: 370-379, July 26, 2007. Web.

[16] Study Group. "A Clinical Trial to Maintain Glycemic Control in Youth with Type 2 Diabetes." *N Engl J Med* 366 (2012): 2247-256. Web.

[17] Nemet, Dan, Sivan Barkan, and Yoram Epstein. "Short- and Long-term Beneficial Effects of a Combined Dietary Behavioral Physical Activity Intervention for the Treatment of Childhood Obesity." *Pediatrics* 115.4 (2005): 2004-172. Web.

[18] Garcia, Ginny, Thankham S. Sunil, and Pedro Hinojosa. "The Fast Food and Obesity Link: Consumption Patterns and Severity of Obesity." *Obesity Surgery* 22.5 (2012): 810-18. Web.

[19] Inagami, Sanae, Deborah A. Cohen, Arleen F. Brown, and Steven M. Asch. "Body Mass Index, Neighborhood Fast Food and Restaurant Concentration, and Car Ownership." *Journal of Urban Health* 86.5 (2009): 683-95. Web.

[20] Taheri, S. "The Link between Short Sleep Duration and Obesity: We Should Recommend More Sleep to Prevent Obesity." *Archives of Disease in Childhood* 91.11 (2006): 881-84. Print.

[21] Ebbeling, C. B., J. F. Swain, and H. A. Feldman. "Effects of Dietary Composition on Energy Expenditure During Weight Loss Maintenance." *JAMA* 307.24 (2012): 2627-634. Print.